150 Survival Lessons:
Useful Tips You Should Know In Order To Survive Everywhere

Disclamer: All photos used in this book, including the cover photo were made available under a Attribution-NonCommercial-ShareAlike 2.0 Generic and sourced from Flickr

Table of content

Survival Communication

Introduction

Survival communication during tough situations is really necessary as without it, you will not be able to get out of tensed situation. Mobile phone communications have a ton of vulnerabilities like being subject to mobile locales which can be influenced in catastrophes like surges and earth tremors, low battery life, and so on, which makes it a poor decision for communication for long-term crises. As specified before, substantial winds and flooding can upset mobile towers and links bringing on the loss of sign like what happened during Hurricane Sandy and many other natural calamities as well. Mobile locales or towers works on AC control only and this can be a major issue when the fundamental force source is upset which is generally the case during trips.

Most mobile towers use generators for reinforcement power supply however generators are the fleeting plan as they require fuel that must be renewed again and again. Mobile phone communication relies on back pull frameworks that are not generally strong since they are wired which can, in any case, be influenced by surges and earth quacks. Mobile phones have a short battery life which would keep going for a day or three. This can be a major issue for long term debacles or emergency since you won't have the capacity to make use of your PDA unless you have a local energy source to back it up.

Mobile phones oblige satellites to build up a steady flag for communication. Shockingly satellites are defenseless against physical assaults, programs, and sunlight based tempests. Whenever force and business lines are down, the best way to have the capacity to interface with the outside world is by utilizing radios as emergency communication gear. Since they don't rely on upon AC force, satellites, or business lines, so they require alternatives to set up a sign for communication.

Chapter 1 – Communication for survival in intense situation

If you get yourself stuck in any disaster and there is no way out then, you must be thinking the way by which you can communicate with your family. Definitely, when you are facing a kind of calamity and there is no one to help you out then you will require something to communicate to your family for sure. In that situation, you cannot just rely on the use of mobile phones. This is because there may be a chance that your mobile battery goes down or may be the place where you reside does not have mobile towers to transmit signals. So, you must look for some kind of alternatives to communicate with your friends and family.

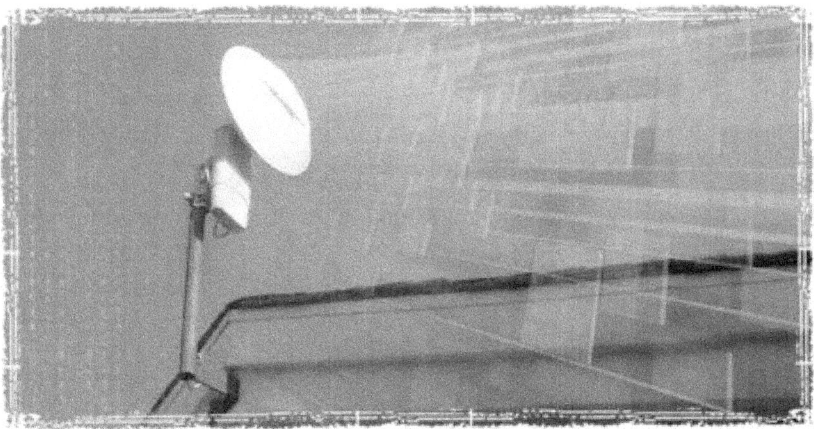

Here, I am going to discuss several ways by which you can communicate with your loved ones and can call them to take you out of that calamity you are facing. Crises which is short-term have demonstrated the impediments of making use of phones to have proper communication with each other. Regardless of the possibility that the towers are operational, they can't deal with the additional move-ment of so many individuals, who attempt to take a few things to get back to some composure of friends and family or help.

How to communicate during a crisis?

During so many occasions which have occurred recently, the services of mobile phones cannot be taken as the most important option for quite a long time. The framework turned out to be genuinely over-burdened on 9/11 so calls failed to be made. 70% of the towers went down during the flood Katrina and were down for a considerable length of time, and most territories haven't been satisfactorily en-hanced throughout the Unites States.

These won't be detached occasions. Try not to believe that since you live in a sub-stantial metropolitan region, you will find yourself more secure. Take a look at a portion of the things that continued during Hurricane Sandy in New York. This will demonstrate that the legislature has a lot of things to manage by simply at-tempting to recover your phone service up so, despite the fact that that was an entirely transient occasion, it brought on a lot of issues.

- Phone correspondence has a great deal of susceptibilities that mark it a pitiable answer for far-reaching or long-lasting crises.

- Substantial airstreams or water overflowing can upset the links between towers, for example, for the duration of Hurricane Sandy.

Mobile towers have need of AC energy to work so in case they don't have a programmed reinforcement framework, they stop. Remember that a wide range of towers are simply celebrated radio wires on the highest points of structures or foothills and reinforcement force, for example, a backup generator is a fleeting plan. Generators entail fuel and that oil must be recharged frequently. In many circumstances, the main reinforcement power which is accessible is a store of batteries that twitch charging as soon as the primary force framework stops.

Back term frameworks that are basically the framework that interfaces or permits flood from external frameworks to the center, regularly include different transporters, aren't generally strong. A great deal of this framework is supported however has been extended to the microwave and different frameworks as well.

Most mobile phones will just remain charged for a couple of days. In case you don't have the local energy to retain it high, when the framework comes move down, you won't have the capacity to converse with it. Mobile phones have need of outposts, that are defenseless against programs, physical assault, or sun oriented tempests. They'll be truly pointless if the countrywide framework goes down because of a digital assault, CME or EMP, that is significantly more probable than you may suspect.

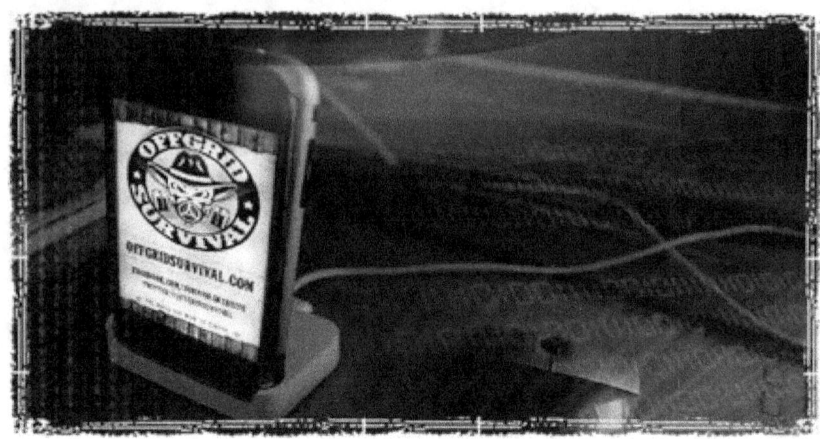

One cool thought that is turning on view is the goTenna mobile phone radio wire framework. Your mobile phone interfaces with it by means of Bluetooth and an application, and the sign is sent and got through a scrambled radio sign. It won't have the capacity to reach to the opposite side of a city however you ought to have the capacity to find your family in case they're in the territory and perhaps speak with others in case they have the framework.

Chapter 2 – How to communicate during worse situations?

There can be so many options that should be taken into consideration by you if you are looking for survival communication. Here are some of the devices which will help you in communication without trouble.

CB radio

Many people developed up viewing the Bear and BJ and they saw every one of the haulers having conversation over the air with one another. CB radio is certainly more accessible during an emergency but they have a lot of restrictions.

According to some, not many individuals are on CB. You may have the capacity to discover somebody in a wagon however even that is harder to discover. The issue isn't only the absence of individuals who utilize it, it's the absence of individuals in your reach that make use of it.

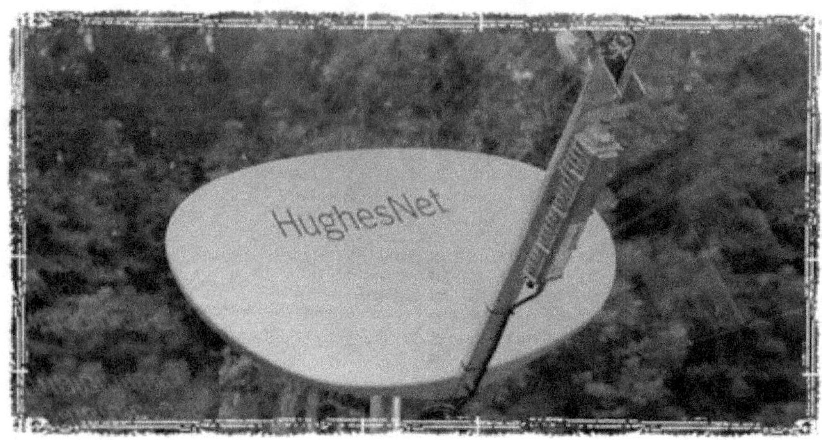

Amongst the enormous reasons your extent is extremely restricted with CB versus different frameworks is that they're constrained to input of 5 watts which is around output of 4 watt. It might be only some dubious thought but additional power results in more unglued. At the regularities that CB transistors utilizes, you can just hope to get somewhere sandwiched between 1 and 10 loads or miles or something like that, contingent upon the landscape. There can be a billion people in the Unites States with their CB's all on the similar network in the meantime, but in case they do not inside reach, you won't talk.

You may imagine that you can simply scribbler into your veal radio and thrust out extra control, however the FCC follows individuals who try to do that in only a couple of cases. Clearly with SHTF, you're not going to truly think around that however rather recall that addition with more energy to transmit. Also, to get more remote doesn't do whatever to benefit you listens to the former person with an ordinary CB transmitter.

Should you opt for satellite phone for an emergency?

In many emergency circumstances, the satellite phones are quite great. The primary issue with them, however, is an expense. They're really very costly. Not just do you need to spend for the phone, you need to recompense for package and minutes. In case you're stranded at some place, it may be justified regardless of the expense.

They don't generally work, however. You should have one with you at all times, and it will come in a hell of convenience. They don't care for wildernesses however-er because of the trees obstructing the satellites and in opposition to what each cracking film appears, they don't work inside a boat like they continued appearing in World War Z.

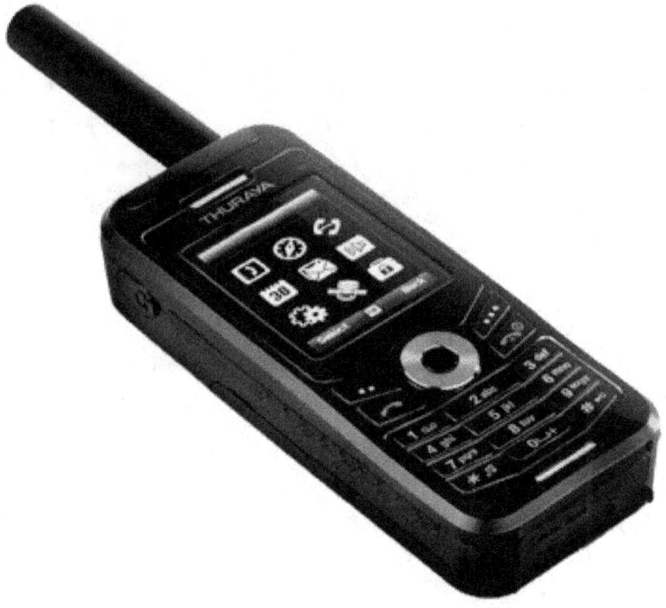

The genuine issue is that it's very improbable that you'd need it in an ordinary family unit so they're only useful for crises and most likely they are not worth the expense. Another enormous issue is that simply like mobile phones, they be determined by on the outposts to have a great capacity so if the outposts quit functioning, the satellite phones will also do the same. Clearly. Sunlight based tempests and CMEs have reserved out satellites previously. They will do it once more.

GMRS radios

For nearby correspondence, MURS radios and GMRS and FRS are truly great. They don't require an FCC permit for MURS and FRS, they're tranquil to operate and simple to be understood. They've basically substituted CB radios for a considerable measure of families. In that capacity, despite the fact that they're a change, they have a ton of the same restriction on force and range.

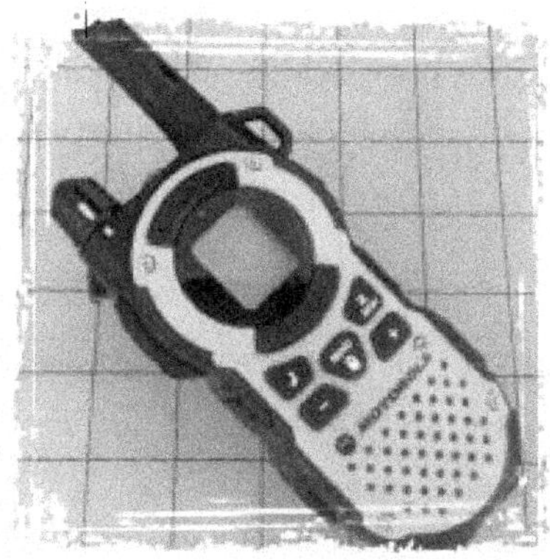

In case you have a genuine GMRS radio, you might possess the capacity to take benefit of a repeater that will extend your reach to conceivably several miles. But, the repeater clearly must run, and you must be within the scope for your radio's repeater to knockout it. GMRS transistors are likewise permitted to work at a higher force than a considerable measure of different radios. You likewise require a permit to make use of GMRS frequencies. Fundamentally, in case you're thinking about one of these radio frameworks to be used in an emergency, you should opt for a genuine GMRS transistor and acquire the license.

The remarkable communication system for emergency cases:

So now that I've given you a few alternatives that you can pick, here I am going to tell you about various other alternatives as well.

Ham transistor is the go-to correspondence framework to be used for basically every emergency system and it is the thing that MARS and ARES both use.

One of the pleasant effects is that a considerable measure of ham transistors can achieve the frequencies of national climate framework. That implies that in case you possess a radio, you can discover what's happening in the range.

Here is an underprivileged of alternative transistor frequencies which you ought to remember when both searching for radios and thinking of your emergency correspondences systems. Just to mollify all the know-it-alls who continue letting you know this rundown is really effective in light of the fact that you can't transmit on them. You should remember that they're valuable to screen in crises regardless of the fact that you can't send anything out, and I needed to make as complete a list as I can make for everybody.

FRS walkie-talkies

FRS radios or family radio service is an intense however short-extended service that you can use to speak with your family within your home or campground. This is a decent choice to add on your emergency survival pack since it is cheap and simple to make use of which implies that, everybody in your group or family can make use of it. FRS radios can likewise speak with GMRS that is General versatile radio service, as they share a few frequencies.

However, FRS two-way radios have their constraints to within its reach extraordinarily. Despite the fact that tests demonstrated that FRS radios can achieve a score of 22 to 36 miles, this is just feasible during ideal conditions which are extremely troublesome during calamities and emergency situation. So FRS radios are best to make use of the place inside your camp, it is still best to make use of all the more effective radios like HAM to get more range and a higher shot of external communication.

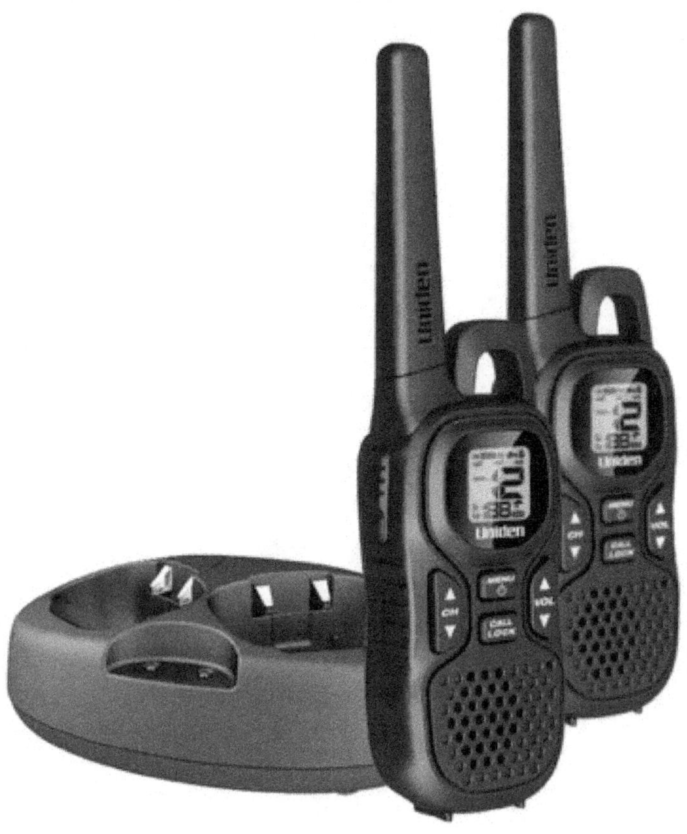

Scanner Radios

A scanner radio is one of the must have radios in your emergency survival kit as it gives you the capacity to listen to other radio transmissions in your general vicinity from various companies like fire divisions, police, emergency vehicle services, government offices, and air. Having a scanner radio during a trip is one of the ideal approaches to reach the world so you may know how to suitably react to the circumstance and for communicating with your family.

Chapter 3 – Survival communication tips

It is true without any doubt that the survival kit will work as the main thing which will make you survived from any of the problems which come to you. The need of survival kits for any family is different as all the families are having different sets of needs which are associated with them. If you want to get ready for any type of emergency situation then this survival kit will also help you in all situation.

Also, when you opt for having survival kits for any of the emergency circumstances which you face, you will also get the option of storing water and its purification tool. It may sometimes happen that you may need some kit which can be personalized by you. So, you can also customize the kit as per you desire without facing any kind of problem.

A proper plan of action along with your customized or even the essential survival kit will help you a lot in surviving from the tough situations along with the assistance to have an adequate supply of water with you as well, as water is a necessary and basic need for keep moving the vehicle of your life.

So many people are of the view that they will not face anything bad so there is no need of having any survival kit with them. But I must tell you here, that this thing is worst to be taken in mind owing to the fact that when it comes to survival, no one knees whenever you will get to need it at any time. It is also a matter of fact that no one can ever be able to get himself prepared for some kind of emergency situation but it is really better to think about to be safe before facing any kind of problem.

The contents which are going to be included in any of the survival kits vary from one place to another. Also, the purpose and location where the survival kit is going to be used will also determine what will be those contents, which are going to be included in that kit.

But, as far as the universality of the survival communication toolkit is concerned, there are some of the contents which are common to all the kits and which are necessary for survival in any kind of situation no matter how severe the situation are. So, you should be very careful about all the things which are common and also, do not forget to keep in mind the extent to which the survival kits may vary from one place to another.

So, just before making your own survival kit, you must be having in your mind about the tools which should be there in order to make your kit completed. You are required to take the proper communication tools with you along with other things which are required. If you are on an outside trip at some place which is at a forest or any mountains, your survival kit must be having some tools, which will help you to stay safe and secure when you are on your journey. You must be having a knife and an ax with you so that you can cut the branches of trees or anything which you require. This will help you in building your shed or any shelter so that you may become able to be secure and safe even if the weather conditions are not so good.

Now, it is not necessary that you should have the knife which is being made by the traditional ways. Anything which can be used as a sharpening tool can be taken as something which resembles knife and which will help you in cutting anything you want. For example, if you are having something to be called as canned food in your survival kit, but you must require having some sharp thing which can be used to cut the can. So, a knife or some sharp thing is a must thing which you require. Along with the cans of tin, the glass and some other things of the same hard material also require having something like a knife to be cut down.

Some more survival communication tips

Repeaters

There are a ton of repeaters in the world that can help you transmit long separations with only a radio. Essentially, a repeater will listen to the small radios in its quick surroundings and afterward impact the sign out for hundreds, or thousands, of miles. Clearly the repeaters should have got the capacity to do this, however, individuals who have repeaters are for the most part upon emergency communication and will have systems for reinforcement power as well.

There are even repeaters that make use of the internet. So in case, you take advantage of a repeater and have been struck in another location, then what you say on your minimal radio will impact out to that point on the opposite side of the world.

Utilizing stealth to work with a novice radio

Since ham radio individuals are cunning parcel and some spots don't permit the use of reception tools, there is an entire sub-sort of approaches to make the receiving wires so they can't be identified. Receiving wires can be made out of flagpoles, stepping stools, wall, railings, and a considerable measure of different things on display. They can likewise be covered up with some other internal things or covers.

The Ham radio group

As I've said, novice radio services are not just innovative and clever, they're extremely tuned in to taking care of the emergency situation. There are a few groups that make use of a ham radio for managing trips or for inquiry and salvage. The greater of the two are Radio Amateur Civil Emergency Service (RACES) and Amateur Radio Emergency Service (ARES).

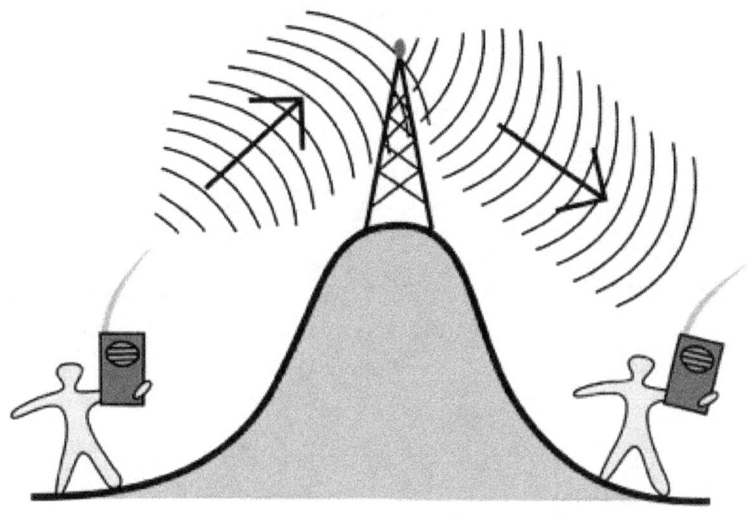

In case you need to start finding out about ham radio as a viable emergency communications framework for you or your family, look at the Prepared Ham Forum. Heaps of accommodating individuals will also be there to assist you in any kind of emergency situation.

Inventive approaches to speak with ham frequencies

With the right gear and some practice, you can undoubtedly get far and wide. What's more, you don't need to really purchase a radio to do it. That is the biggest aspect regarding learning and utilizing ham radio. You can actually make a working radio out of scrap. There will dependably be a scrap. You will dependably have the capacity to make a radio.

Notwithstanding the plenty of ham radio hardware and data accessible, a great premise of the hypothesis can make them converse with individuals regardless of the possibility that all power and gadgets are taken out. Here are a few case of what you can do with a small information.

In the case of a helicopter protection, most pilots will attempt to have land as a first choice. If a sufficiently extensive clearing is accessible than adequate size will rely on the ground, height, wind conditions, and ability of the pilot, a clearing of no less than 80 feet is the thing that generally require. Attempt and position yourself with your back to the wind-confronting the clearing so you're at the 12 to 3 clock position. After it lands, sit tight for salvage workforce to come to you, don't head out to the helicopter, when force is diminished, the rotors can wind up brought down to a point where they can execute a normal tallness individual particularly in case you are up at the slope of the helicopter.

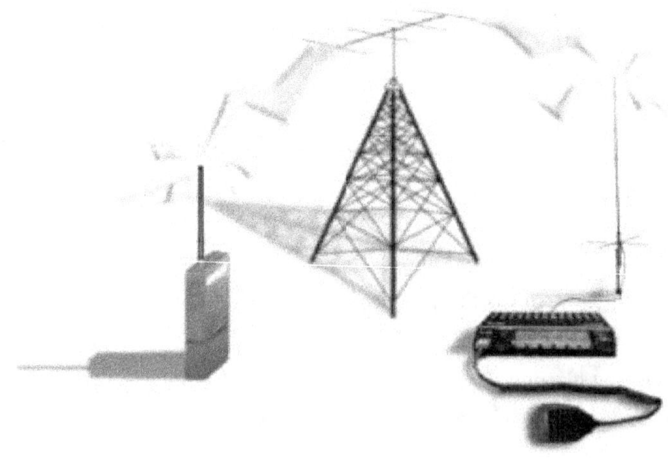

Since weight influences fuel limit which thus influences range and time of flight, don't hope to take your pack or tool with you. In the occasion, the group chooses to bring down a crane or bushel, by and large, a rescuer will ride it down. Try not to attempt and help, particularly abstain from attempting to get the crate or link before it has an opportunity to touch the ground at any rate. The rotors can get the electricity produced via friction over long separations and touching a link or wicker bin before it grounds can give you a stun.

Chapter 4 – How to get rescued by survival communication?

Calling for help or getting protected in an emergency situation is not something the vast majority of us need to do. But rather by investing enough energy outside will give you chances that are you'll encounter some sort of emergency. With regards to making use of your mobile phone and getting safeguarded, here are the tips you can take after, that will help rescuers discover you rapidly, help them, and get you out securely. A snappy salvage expands the chances of survival and can lessen the introduction to safeguarding the parties. Communication and flagging assume an essential part in proficient wild protects. Here are a few things to be considered.

Telling somebody about your plan is imperative. Before you leave for your trip, let somebody know your normal return time, trail or course, destination, auto type and plate number, fundamental tools you'll have, your mobile phone number and bearer, and different names and data related to you. At times, you can likewise portray the color of your tent and coat, and rundown supplies.

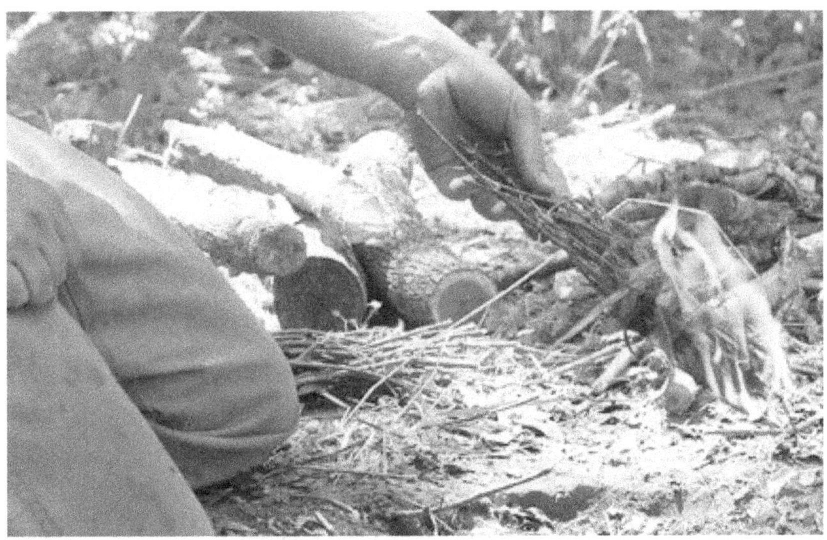

Although, some spots won't have a mobile network accessible in the far off places, the scope is expanding and in so many situations of crises, mobile phones are the most widely recognized method for starting salvage for climbers and explorers. You ought to switch off your phone or radio in case you have one to monitor batteries till you are prepared to make use of it. In cool situations attempt and keep your communication tool near your body to keep it warm and also to preserve the battery life between layers of clothing items. Most new phones consequently settle your area when you make an emergency call, this isn't generally ensured and you can find a way to offer assistance.

A. Prior to your excursion initiate your phones programmed area setting which empowers E911 to ascertain your position.

B. Turn on your phone once per day before an emergency for around 5 minutes, when fueled up phones check in with the closest tower. This should be done regardless of the fact that there is an insufficient sign to make a call, it can be sufficient to leave an electronic trail.

C. Radios and most mobile phones work disconnected from the net of site significance, for example, slopes, mountains, or overwhelming tree spread can obstruct the signals. Satellite phones require an unhindered perspective of the sky. To make an emergency call, higher open areas will give the best flag. So you are required to hold your phone at a manageable distance and pivot around to locate the best group. When you locate the best spot, come back to that spot for future calls.

- Consider what data you'll have to pass on to the emergency service provider. Dial the number of the emergency individual before your emergency contact. Stay quiet, at the request, express your name, your area with however many subtle elements as can be allowed.

- In case, you don't have the foggiest idea about your area depicting encompassing area elements then last known unmistakable focus on the area will likewise offer assistance. Let them know your emergency and individuals included, type of hardware, the amount of food items and fuel you have and the color of the tent, rucksack, garments, and so on, including your emergency contacts data.

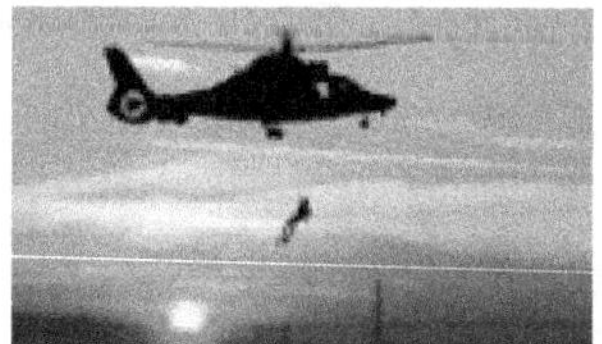

Notice your plan of activity stay put, attempt and exit, set up portable shelter, and assemble a fire, and so on. Before hanging up, let them know you'll turn off your phone and play Judas five minutes before, then look for the highest point of consistently or two, unless told generally by the 911 administrator. Take after some other directions that have been given.

- In case you don't have enough groups to support but a spotty sign, it's conceivable to get an instant message out regardless of the possibility that you can't get a call through. Most emergency services aren't set up to get instant messages so make use of your emergency contact. In case you benefited an occupation of pre-outing communication you'll have the capacity to keep your content short, they'll know who it's originating from and right now have fundamental data.

To flag others material can be regular and you can make use of sticks, rocks, soil, shadows, manmade garments, packs, tents, space covers or both. The vital thing to recall is to take after the class standard for ground to Air signals. "C" remains for Contrast, you perform this with shading that differences the environment. This can be a dark shadow against white snow which can be done by borrowing a trench or Orange tent over green vegetation. The "L" remains for the area, you need an open range that can be seen from various bearings and is near to your own zone.

"A" stands for Angularity, the straighter your lines and more honed your corners are, the better it is. There are not many common 90 degree corners in nature so having them in a sign will get a rescuers attention. "S" remains for Size, the greater your sign the better. S remains for shape, there aren't an excessive number of straight corners or 90-degree twists in nature so having a sign with straight lines and sharp corners will emerge more. The state of your sign can likewise convey data to an air group. A huge implies that you require help. The later X tells the team that you have been harmed, and then you can make use of vast bolts to impart the bearing of travel in case you're leaving a signed zone.

- Development additionally gets the attention, you can perform this with lively arm waves or a shirt toward the end of a shaft. The shirt will likewise have the advantage of informing the helicopter group of the heading of the wind as they have to confront into the wind to make a lift for landing and taking off. A legitimate work makes use of sign mirror that will be spotted to about 100 miles.

- Space covers, aluminum foil, watches, and anything which sparkles can likewise be made out of it. During the evening flares, headlamp (light), and chemical sticks work best. Three sign are light and simple to pack are a sign mirror, shriek, and compound stick. Different things can likewise work assign materials.

Fire signs are one of the best strategies for flagging salvage. The two fundamental issues are bringing on woods fires and the time window between getting the fire to deliver enough smoke to be seen and airship passing. Care must be taken to clear the encompassing vegetation and set up the ground for a fire. Another issue can be the individuals who do not distinguish the fire as a sign.

To fabricate a sign fire, you should first set up the site. Locate an open area near your camp or where you'll invest the majority of your energy. Clear the fire zone, scratching the ground to exposed earth, and broaden it out no less than 15 feet. Prep the kindling with every phase of wood put in a log lodge design with small pieces at the base and bigger wood toward the top.

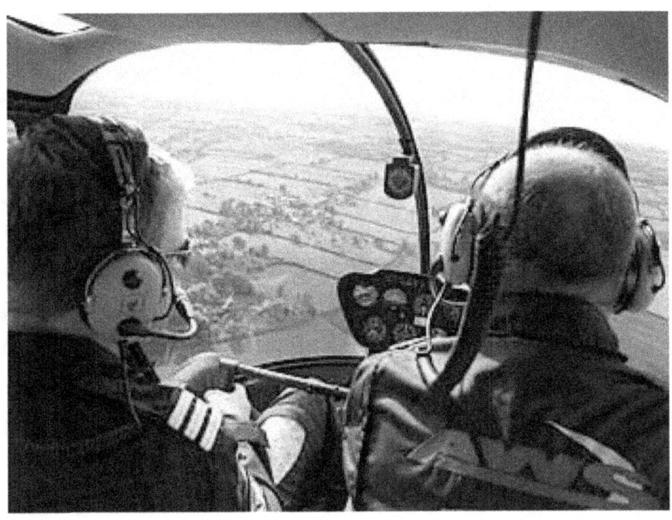

Close to the top you ought to have one to three feet of fuel, and green material including pine limbs, branches, grass, leaves. It creates more smoke than dead dry material. The fire burning material and fuel ought to be dry and dead. Having the green stuff on top will keep the kindling dry at the base. Have a tender close-by and keep dry. When you first hear an airplane or realize that safeguard is in the general zone or fast approaching begin the fire. Once you have waist high flares add green material as expected to keep delivering the smoke.

Conclusion

It is really a matter of fact that everyone feels contented and secure in one's own house. No one is willing to leave one's home or no one will want to have a home which is not protected by the security locks and other things like this. No one will really want to have his/her family in an unprotected environment where there are no locks on the door. It is just like as if you are not having the survival kit with you when you need it the most no matter wherever you are. God forbade, if any of the natural tragedy comes, then your essential survival kit will definitely help you in surviving even in a bad situation. Survival communication comes out to be necessary when you are at trip or may be when you are facing a critical situation.

Survival Cookbook

Introduction

Are you preparing yourself for the most unfavorable circumstances? What would happen if a natural disaster strikes down and you're left alone with very little to carry on? For this very reason, you have to be prepared. If you are a professional prepper, this book is just right for you. Just add this book to your prepping stuff and you'd be able to survive all the tough conditions.

The recipes given in this book are simple and really easy to understand. In times where you have to survive and fight a battle against catastrophes, this book would help you feel like home. These recipes are not only easy and just what a prepper needs, they are really delicious too. You'd not feel you have a survival problem.

In this book, I am sharing 20 recipes that are tasty and what is the best thing about these recipes is that they can be kept in a mason jar for longer periods of time. For, who knows how long you will have to survive and how long would it take someone to come at your rescue. The food that you'd make using these recipes could be preserved and kept for times you have nothing to eat to keep your life going.

Doing the Stuff of confidence requires significant investment, assets, tools, and other things as well. More critical than any of these is the action you take. With just twenty four hours in a day, you can't generally trek to your own space in the forested areas to practice wild basic instincts. Tumultuous calendars and time requirements consume your accessibility. There is no better approach to hang out with your friends and family than to acquaint them with outside independence abilities in a controlled setting.

I have chosen these recipes that are to be made in mason jars because in times where you're alone and you need to survive, you should be able to preserve food for long. Because you are not sure when help would come and it might even take a long period of time before you are rescued so you have to be sure you have preserved enough food for a long period of time.

The capacity to make fire under any condition is basic thing to be done during survival. With How to Build a prepping there are numerous systems to assemble a fire; a fire drill, seething plants and trees, daylight, striking shake that contains iron, for example, rock, and obviously matches and lighters. Fire craft is the capacity to make, control, and utilize fire to help in one's survival. Another basic aptitude in Prepping is the capacity to transfer fire, normally via burning or heating coal in some type of dry sage grass to keep it seething.

There are a total of 20 recipes that you'd learn to make which can be preserved and kept for future use. For when you have to survive, it is not just the present you should be worried about, the future should be taken care of too.

Chapter 1 – Survival Food Storage

If you are a want to-be survivor or a prepper and you have no idea where to start, I'll guide you through that in this chapter. Before anything, the first thing you should do is to store food. Because to make use of the 20 recipes that I've shared in this book, you have to be sure you have almost everything that you need with you and the amount of all that should also be enough to keep you going for a long time. Getting better prepped for unfavorable circumstances doesn't mean you're a pessimist. It means that you're wise and you are thinking about your family and your survival in adverse conditions for who knows when could that happen? So, where to start with storing enough food to help you survive for a long while.

Survival tips envelop a few primitive aptitudes to shape your general surroundings and meet your survival needs. Recall, prepping shows you how to do every one of different things with only a basic tool and the learning in your mind. Each of these prepping aptitudes have numerous littler subsets of undertakings and capacities that make them up.

As should be obvious there is a long way to go. While turning into a prepping expert can take quite a while and without any doubt, there are so many little abilities that can be immediately figured out how to kick you off. Moreover, a part of the more basic abilities like making cordage and branches have numerous uses and can be connected to more than one control. At it is the most basic level of prepping, here is the specialty of going out into the forested areas and getting by just with the clothes on your back and an edged tool. About each ability and most prepping activities utilize a prepping device to make your work simpler.

Steps involved in storing survival food

Let's have a look at how you can store enough amount of food to help you survive before the circumstances come back to normal,

1.   *Planning:*

First thing to do anything is to plan. You cannot just go on and start doing something. You have to make a plan first. This is not the easiest of all the steps. Going to the market and buying stuff is easier but what to buy and in what quantity and from where etc. these require certain decisions to be made. This step is mostly ignore but trust me, you want to do this. So planning is the first and the most critical step involved in storing food.

2.   *Buying:*

So after you've made a plan, go out there and start buying. This should be simple. Get a list of food items to buy, grab your wallet and drive to the market and buy all the stuff.

3.   *Preserving:*

The third step is to preserve food. This step is really important. Now you have to make sure that you preserve the food long enough so that it can be eaten when you want to eat it. Try to get things that can be preserved for at least three years.

4.   *Organizing:*

This is really important that you keep all the food in an organized way. Keep everything separate and in an orderly manner in the storage room.

5.   *Eating:*

This is the best part, of course. For this I've 20 really good recipes for you in the upcoming chapters of this book. You would love each and every recipe.

Now that you have known what are the steps you need to take to store food for prepping. Now let's take a look at how you can store different food items.

6.   *Canning:*

This is a traditional method to preserve food for long periods of times. This involves partially cooking the food to kill any germs or bacteria, adding additives like sugar syrup etc. cleaning the cans or glass jars, drying them and filling them with the food items and then sealing them to store for a long period of time.

7.   *Drying:*

This is probably the easiest way of preserving food. This requires no real efforts. It is known that bacteria and mold grow in moisture. So rest assured, you could keep the food you dry for long span of time and without fearing that it will rot or catch bacteria.

8.   *Salt curing:*

This is an old method which was used to preserve meat for long time. Salt helps keep the meat safe from bacteria because bacteria cannot survive more than 10% of concentration of salt in something. You can rub a mixture of sugar and salt on meat and keep it tightly shut in a pot or jar and keeping it somewhere the temperature is cool.

9.   *Refrigeration:*

This the very famous and very common way of preserving food. Keeping beef, mutton, poultry, cooked food and other items in a refrigerator keeps them safe for a long period of time by keeping the food frozen or cold.

Chapter 2 – 10 Delicious Prepping Recipes for All Seasons in Mason Jars

You have everything kept in your storage to help you survive during circumstances that are adverse. Now you'd need some recipes that would make you feel normal and happy even in times of distress. Let's have a look at some of these recipes,

1) ALMOND MILK & HONEY PORRIDGE:

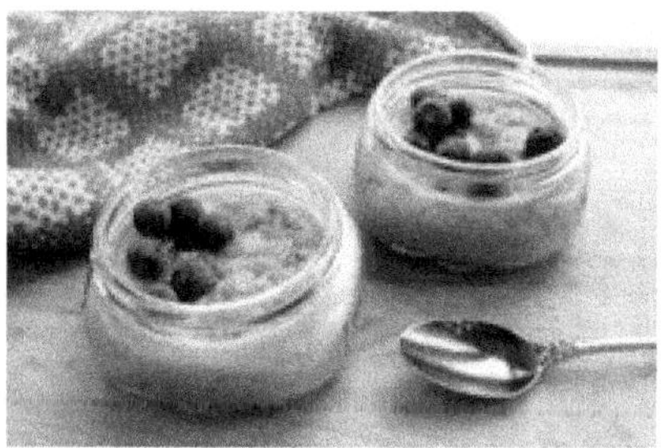

http://photos2.demandstudios.com/DM-Resize/www.livestrong.com/ls_images/recipes/00000/45/77/0/almond-milk-honey-porridge-17754.jpg?w=280&h=280&keep_ratio=1

This is a very simple but nutritious and satisfying recipe that you would be able to make in just 15 minutes. This recipe would serve 3 persons. You would need the following ingredients,

- Cooked Quinoa (2 cups)

- Ground Nutmeg (2 pinches)

- Unsweetened almond milk (1 and a half cup)

- Natural Almond Butter (1 and half tbsp.)

- Vanilla extract (1 and half tbsp.)

- Sea Salt (1 pinch)

What to do?

1. Blend quinoa and one cup almond milk in a blender until mixed well. Pour this mixture in a pot and cook over medium heat. Take the remaining half cup of almond milk and mix it in the mixture using a stirrer. Add vanilla essence, nutmeg and sea salt into the mixture and cook until bubbles start appearing. Add almond butter and stir.

2. Take mason jars and pour the mixture into them and garnish them with fresh berries if you like.

2) CHICKEN CURRY SALAD WITH GREENS:

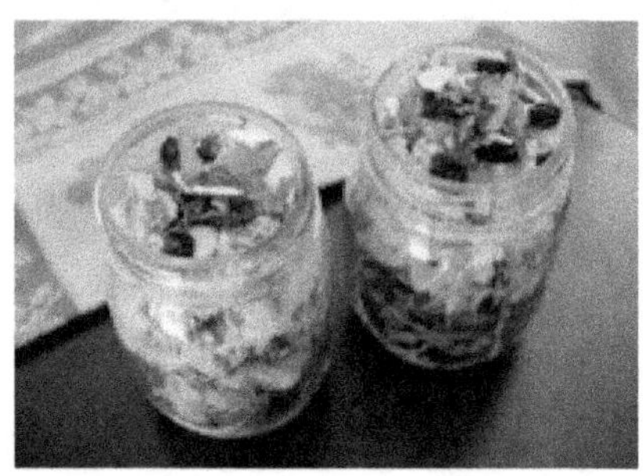

http://photos2.demandstudios.com/DM-Resize/www.livestrong.com/ls_images/recipes/00000/55/77/0/chicken-curry-salad-greens-17755.jpg?w=280&h=280&keep_ratio=1

This is a creamy chicken salad that is a very good source of protein for your body. It would take almost an hour for you to complete this recipe. This recipe serves 7 people. The ingredients are,

- Skinless Chicken Breast (3 pieces)

- Mayonnaise (1/3 cup)

- Low-fat Greek yogurt (1/3 cup)

- Curry Powder (1 serving)

- Sea salt (half tsp)

- Ground Black Pepper (1 dash)

- 1 Grated carrot

- 1 chopped celery stalk

- Raisins (1/2 cup)

- Unsalted Dry Toasted Slivered Almonds (1/4 cup)

- Arugula (4 cups)

What to do?

- Preheat your oven at 375 degrees. Take a large baking tray and cover it with tinfoil. Bake the chicken in the over for almost 45 minutes. The chicken should be thoroughly cooked and light golden brown in color. Let it cool down for some time. Take the chicken and shred the meat.

- Whisk mayo, Greek yogurt, salt and pepper in a small bowl. Add 1 tbsp.. of curry powder to the mixture and mix it well. You can add more curry powder according to your taste.

- Take a bowl and put the shredded chicken, grated carrot and chopped celery in it. Pour the curry sauce that you've made into the bowl and mix everything gently. Put raisins and almonds in the mixture too. Take a mason jar and make a layer of arugula at the bottom and then pour the curry salad above it. Your recipe is ready!

3) FRUIT SOUP WITH TOASTED NUTS:

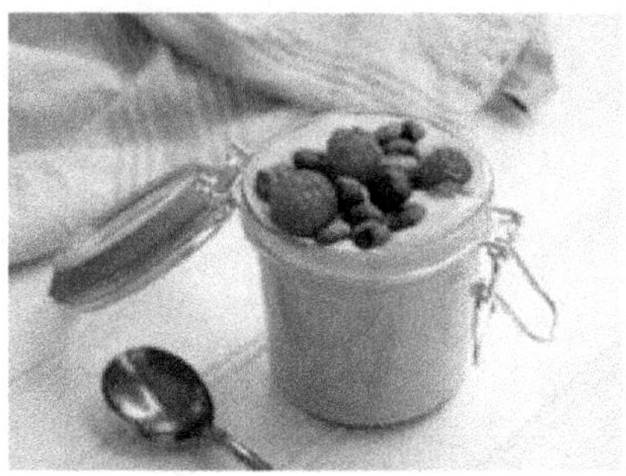

http://photos2.demandstudios.com/DM-Resize/www.livestrong.com/ls_images/recipes/00000/16/77/0/fruit-soup-toasted-nuts-17761.jpg?w=280&h=280&keep_ratio=1

This recipe is full of tasty Greek yogurt combined with fruit. This recipe is perfect for a strong protein breakfast. Takes just 15 minutes to make and serves 2 people. The ingredients include,

- Shelled Pistachios (2 tbsp.)

- low-fat Greek yogurt (1 and a half cup)

- Frozen Mixed Berries Frozen (1 cup)

- Vanilla extract (1 1/4 tsp)

- Agave nectar (2 tbsp.)

- Ground nutmeg (1 pinch)

- Unsweetened Almond Milk (1/2 cup)

- Raspberries (1/4 cup)

What to do?

If you want you can roast the nuts at 350 degrees for 5 minutes. Take Greek yogurt, berries, vanilla, and agave nectar, nutmeg and almond milk and blend them well in a blender. Make sure the result is creamy and smooth. Store in a Mason jar and put lots of fruit on top of it. Serve with a spoon when you want to eat.

4) CHICKEN APPLE AND CASHEW SALAD:

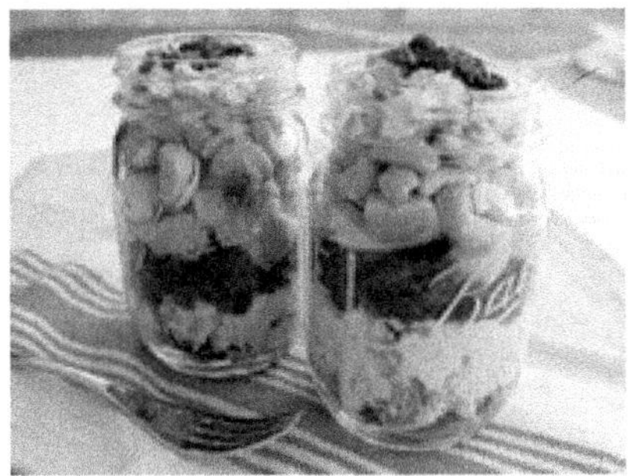

http://photos2.demandstudios.com/DM-Resize/www.livestrong.com/ls_images/recipes/00000/85/77/0/chicken-apple-cashew-salad-17758.jpg?w=280&h=280&keep_ratio=1

A perfect balanced lunch with carbohydrates, proteins and fat. This recipe would take an hour to make and will serve 8 people. Following are the ingredients,

- Skinless Chicken Breast (3 pieces)

- Mayonnaise (1/3 cup)

- Low-fat Greek yogurt (1/3 cup)

- A medium celery stalk

- Sea Salt (1/2 tsp)

- Ground Black Pepper

- Chopped fresh Thyme (1/2 tsp)

- Chopped Green Apple (3 serving)

- Dry Roasted Unsalted Cashews (1/4 cup)

- Dried Cranberries (1/3 cup)

What to do?

- Preheat your oven at 375 degrees. Take a large baking tray and cover it with tinfoil. Bake the chicken in the over for almost 45 minutes. The chicken should be thoroughly cooked and light golden brown in color. Let it cool down for some time. Take the chicken and shred the meat.

- Whisk mayo, Greek yogurt, salt and pepper in a small bowl. Put in celery, celery leaves and thyme and stir well.

- Take a mason jar and make a layer of arugula at the bottom and then pour the chicken salad above it. Put green apple, cashews and cranberries on top. Enjoy!

5) OVERNIGHT APPLE PIE PROTEIN OATS:

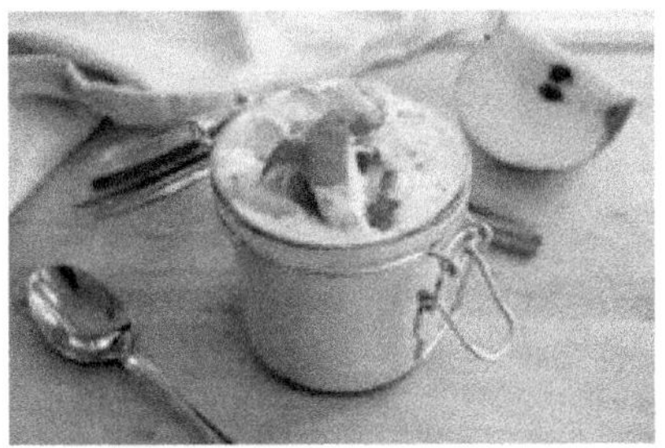

http://photos2.demandstudios.com/DM-Resize/www.livestrong.com/ls_images/recipes/00000/37/77/0/overnight-apple-pie-protein-oats-17773.jpg?w=280&h=280&keep_ratio=1

Another absolutely nutritious and yummy recipe. This recipe would take you 10 minutes to make. It serves 2 persons. You would need,

- 1 Second Cooking Spray

- Chopped apple (1 serving)

- Cinnamon (1 pinch)

- Proto Whey Vanilla (2 scoops)

- Low-fat Greek yogurt (2/3 cup)

- Vanilla extract (1 tsp)

- Ground Nutmeg (2 dash)

- Ground Allspice (2 dash)

- Sea Salt (1 pinch)

- Unsweetened Almond Milk (3/4 cup)

- Old Fashioned Oats (2/3 cup)

- Chia seeds (2 tbsp.)

What to do?

1. Take a small pan and spray it with cooking oil. Sauté apple until it's soft. Add cinnamon and set it aside.

2. Blend protein powder, Greek yogurt, and vanilla, nutmeg, and allspice, salt and almond milk in a blender until mixed well.

3. Mix the oats and chia seeds and stir them. Put them in mason jars.

4. Put sautéed apple on top of it. Stir it and keep it in the refrigerator overnight.

6) TURKEY BASIL MEATBALLS:

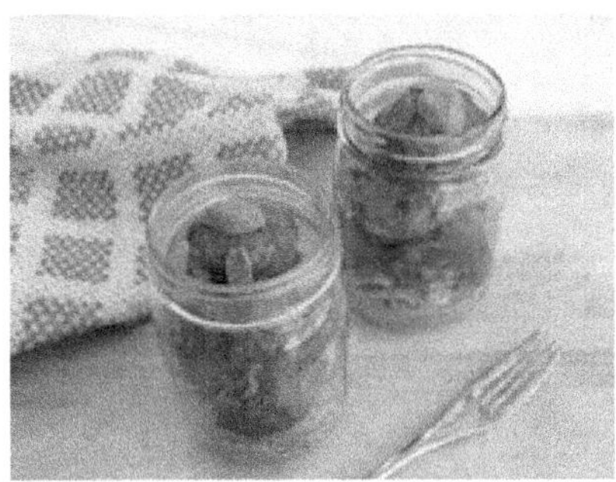

http://photos2.demandstudios.com/DM-Resize/www.livestrong.com/ls_images/recipes/00000/46/77/0/turkey-basil-meatballs-2-17764.jpg?w=280&h=280&keep_ratio=1

Meatballs are about fat and calories. A complete meal. This recipe would be complete in 50 minutes. Total servings: 6. let's check out the ingredients,

- 1 second Cooking Spray

- Grated onion (1/2)

- Minced garlic cloves (4)

- Fresh chopped Basil (1/4 cup)

- Beaten Egg (1)

- Worcestershire Sauce (1 tbsp.)

- All Natural Tomato Paste (2 tsp)

- Pecorino Grated Romano Cheese (4 tbsp.)

- Sea Salt (1/2 tsp)

- Pure Ground Black Pepper (1 serving)

- 92% lean Ground Turkey (20 oz)

- Gluten Free Bread Crumbs (1/3 cup)

- Organic Tomato Sauce (28 oz)

What to do?

1. Preheat your oven to 325 degrees. Take a large baking sheet and spray it with cooking spray.

2. Take a medium size bowl and whisk together onion, garlic, Worcestershire sauce, tomato paste, fresh basil, egg, cheese, salt and pepper until they are mixed well. Take the turkey and mix it with bread crumbs with your hands. Make sure you don't over-mix them. If the mixture is still wet, add some more bread crumbs.

3. Make 24 balls with your hands. Bake these balls for 20 minutes almost. Turn the balls halfway through the baking. Make sure you don't overcook the balls.

4. Meanwhile, make pasta according to the directions on the box.

5. Take a pot and heat the sauce in it over medium heat.

6. Make a layer of pasta in the Mason jar and put the meatballs and sauce above it. Garnish with basil.

7) UPSIDE DOWN CEREAL AND PROTEIN MILK:

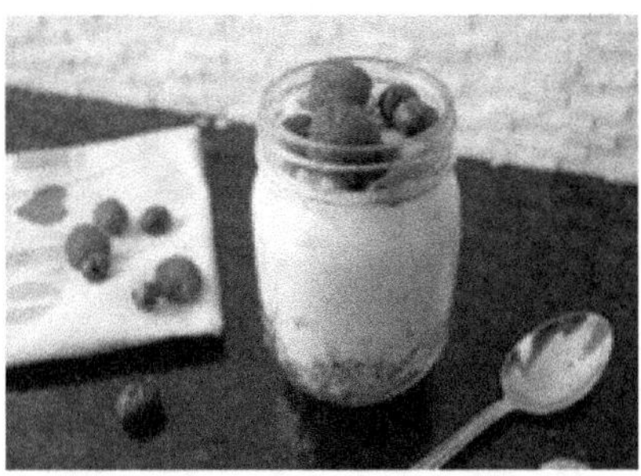

http://photos2.demandstudios.com/DM-Resize/www.livestrong.com/ls_images/recipes/00000/26/77/0/upside-down-cereal-protein-milk-17762.jpg?w=280&h=280&keep_ratio=1

This recipe would help you boost up your metabolism. It would only take 5 minutes to be ready. Serves one person. The ingredients are,

- Gluten Free Sunrise Crunchy Vanilla (2/3 cup)

- Low-fat Greek yogurt (1 cup)

- Proto Whey, Vanilla Crème (1/2 scoops)

- Vanilla extract (1 tsp)

- Unsweetened Almond Milk (1/3 cup)

What to do?

1. Take a mason jar and pour cereal in it.

2. Blend Greek yogurt, protein powder, vanilla and almond milk in a blender until its smooth.

3. Before you serve it, pour protein milk on the cereal. Garnish it with fresh berries if you like.

8) BACON & EGGS IN A JAR:

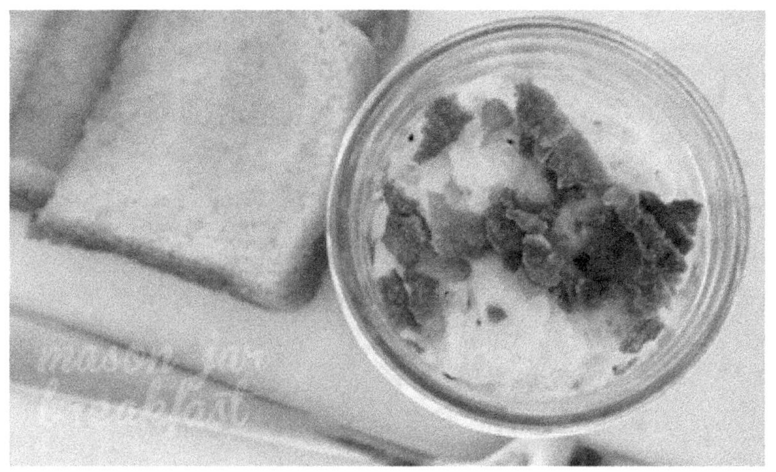

http://www.masonjarbreakfast.com/wp-content/uploads/2014/04/bacon-top.png

An instant recipe that would take only 5 minutes! The ingredients are,

- Bacon

- Eggs (2)

- Shredded Cheese

- Fresh Spinach

- Dash Salt & Pepper

What to do?

1. Take a bowl and mix eggs, spinach, salt & pepper and cheese together.

2. Take a mason jar and pour the mixture in it.

3. Cook the mixture in the microwave oven for 2 minutes at leasts.

4. Garnish with some additional cheese & bacon crumbles.

9) ACAI BANANA BERRY SMOOTHIE:

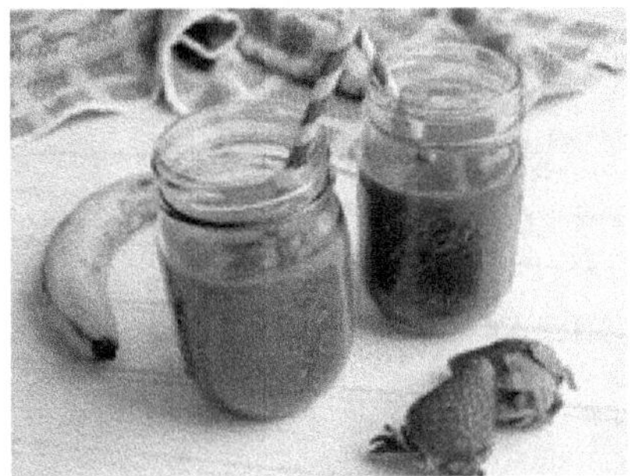

http://photos2.demandstudios.com/DM-Resize/www.livestrong.com/ls_images/recipes/00000/35/77/0/acai-banana-berry-smoothie-2-17753.jpg?w=280&h=280&keep_ratio=1

This smoothie is perfect for you when your blood sugar level drops. Takes 5 minutes to make, the ingredients include,

- Unsweetened almond milk (one and half cup)

- 1 Banana (medium)

- Chopped strawberries (1/2 cup)

- Acai powder (2 tbsp.)

- Proto Whey, Vanilla Cream (4 scoops)

What to do?

Take a blender and place almond milk, banana, strawberries, acai powder and Proto Whey Vanilla Cream in it until the mixture is blended completely. Add ice and blend until smooth and creamy.

10) SHRIMP AND VEGETABLE SALAD WITH COCONUT PEANUT SAUCE:

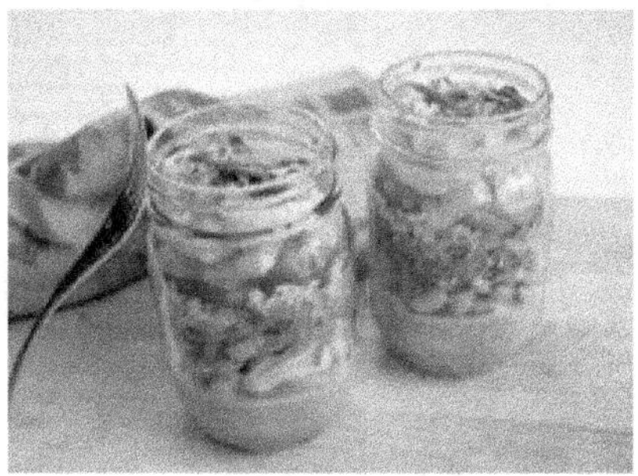

http://photos2.demandstudios.com/DM-Resize/www.livestrong.com/ls_images/recipes/00000/67/77/0/shrimp-vegetable-salad-coconut-peanut-sauce-17776.jpg?w=280&h=280&keep_ratio=1

This recipe would only take 25 minutes to make. Serves 4 people. The ingredients are,

- Light Coconut Milk Light (1/4 cup)

- All Natural Peanut Butter (1/4 cup)

- Low-sodium soy sauce (2 tbsp.)

- Agave nectar (1 tbsp.)

- Sriracha sauce (2 tsp)

- Minced garlic cloves (2)

- Raw Lime Juice (1 tbsp.)

- Cooked Medium Shrimp (16 oz)

- Organic Edamame (1 cup)

- 1 chopped red bell pepper

- 1 chopped yellow bell pepper

- 1 grated carrot

- Cooked Brown Basmati Rice (1 cup)

- Fresh chopped cilantro (1/4 cup)

What to do?

1. Whisk together the first 7 ingredients. Taste it and if you like you can add more lime juice.

2. Take a mason jar and layer it with coconut peanut sauce. Add shrimps, edamame, peppers, cilantro, carrots and brown rice on top

3. Shake the Mason jar when you want to eat it.

Chapter 3 – 10 Delicious Recipes for Summer in Mason Jars

In this chapter, I have 10 very nice recipes that you could make and eat all summers. Let's start!!

1) BLUEBERRY PANCAKE IN A JAR:

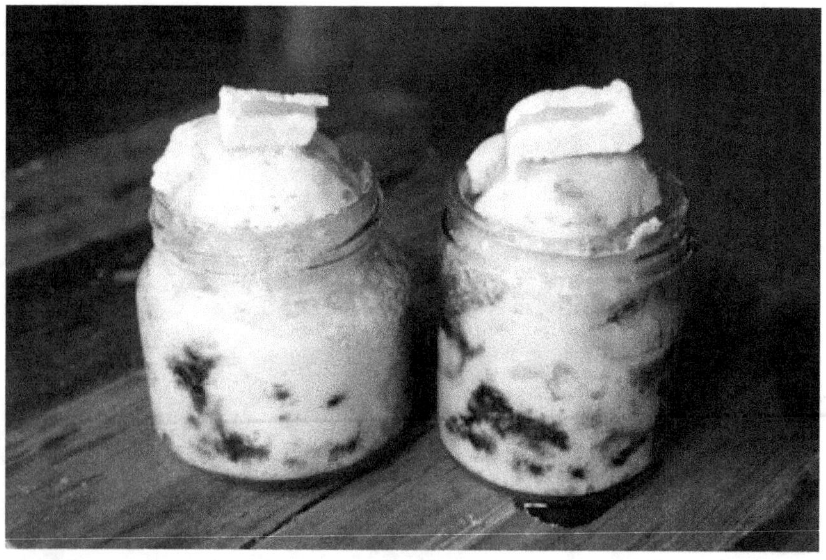

https://boyandtherabbit.files.wordpress.com/2012/07/blog-111.jpg?w=620

This is an incredible recipe for summers. You'll need the following ingredients,

- Flour (1 cup)

- Baking powder (1 tbsp.)

- Organic sugar (2 tbsp.)

- Melted vegan margarine (2 tbsp.)

- Nut milk (3/4 cup)

- Blueberries

What to do?

1. Take a small bowl and mix flour, baking powder and sugar in it. Add melted margarine and milk and stir.

2. Take mason jars and place blueberries at the bottom and fill the jars with the mixture. Pancake will rise after it's cooked. Microwave the jars for 1-1:30 minutes depending on the size of the jars. Let the jars cool. Then put margarine, blueberries and syrup on top. Enjoy!

2) STRAWBERRY & CHOCOLATE YOGURT PARFAIT:

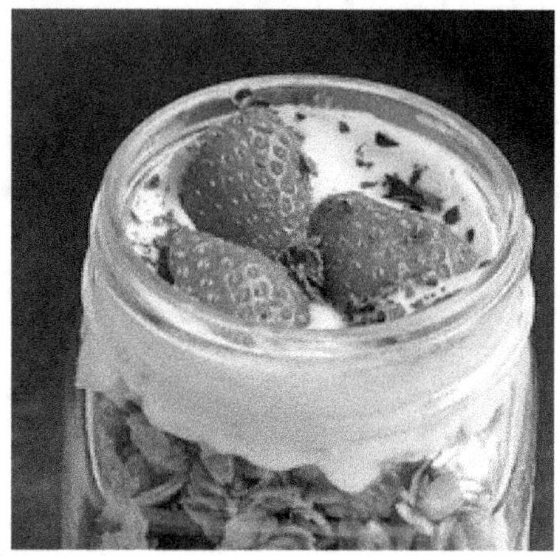

https://img.buzzfeed.com/buzzfeed-static/static/2014-07/7/18/enhanced/web-dr10/grid-cell-32443-1404770627-20.jpg

- For this extremely delicious recipe, you'd need the following ingredients,

- Greek whole yogurt (1/2 - 3/4 cup)

- Granola (2/3 cup)

- 5-6 organic strawberries

- Organic chocolate bar (1-2 oz)

What to do?

1. Layer your parfait with 1/4 cup of yogurt.

2. Put 1/3 cup of granola on top.

3. Put pieces of chocolates and 2 strawberries sliced up on the top.

4. Repeat this procedure and put yogurt on top.

5. Garnish with strawberries and chocolate.

3) WHEAT BERRY APPLE SALAD:

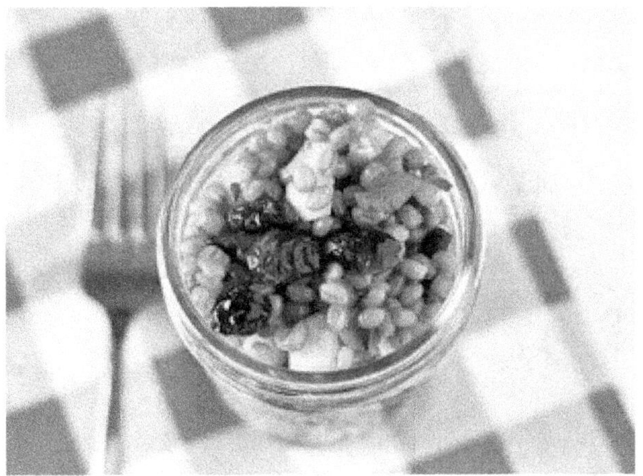

https://img.buzzfeed.com/buzzfeed-static/static/2014-07/7/18/enhanced/web-dr06/grid-cell-20775-1404770869-29.jpg

Let's check out how you can make this yummy recipe,

- Wheat Berry Apple Salad

- Cooked wheat berries

- Chopped organic granny smith apple

- Dried cranberries

- Minced scallions or sweet onion

- Chopped Parsley

- Lemon juice

- Balsamic vinegar

- Olive oil

What to do?

Take all these ingredients and mix them in a bowl. Put the bowl aside. Take lemon juice, balsamic vinegar and olive oil in a bowl and whisk it until mixed completely. Mix these mixture with the salad.

4) SHRIMP FETA SALAD:

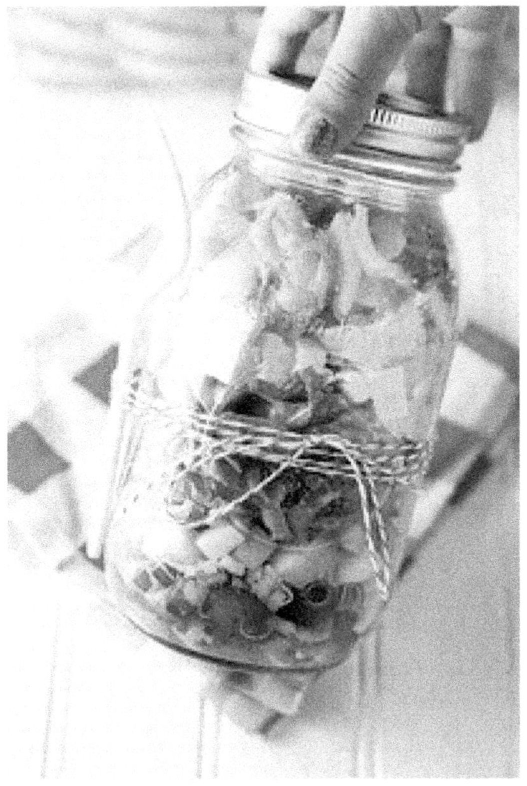

https://img.buzzfeed.com/buzzfeed-static/static/2014-07/7/18/enhanced/web-dr06/grid-cell-25423-1404771284-7.jpg

This yummy summer salad would be a treat for you!

- Dressing of your liking

- Chopped avocado (2 tbsp.)

- 8 grape tomatoes

- Chopped red onion (1 tbsp.)

- Chopped cucumber (2 tbsp.)

- Romaine lettuce

- Baby spinach

- Chopped feta (2 tbsp.)

- 6-8 cooked shrimp

- 1 chopped boiled egg

- 2 slices of chopped cooked bacon

What to do?

Take a mason jar, make layers of all the above ingredients starting with the dressing of your own choice. Done!!

5) CAPRESE SALAD IN MASON JAR:

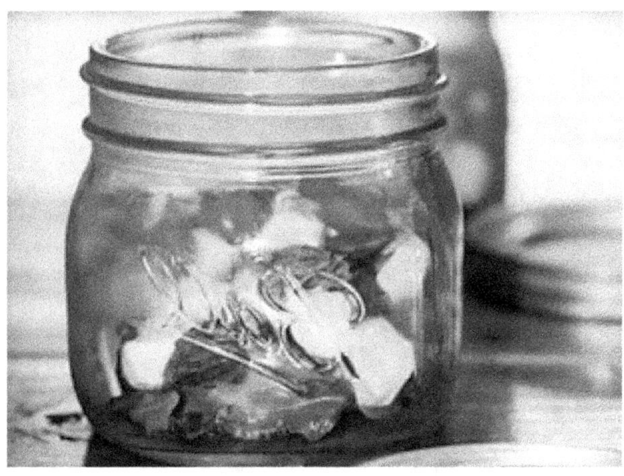

https://img.buzzfeed.com/buzzfeed-static/static/2014-07/7/18/enhanced/web-dr05/grid-cell-1507-1404771206-14.jpg

Ingredients for this recipe are,

- Arugula (2 cups)

- Green basil leaves only (1/2 cup)

- Purple basil leaves (1/2 cup)

- Cherry tomatoes (1/2 cup)

For the dressing:

- Olive oil (1/2 cup)

- Balsamic vinegar (1/2 tbsp.)

- Honey

- Maldon salt

- Black pepper (Cracked)

What to do?

1. Make layers of all the ingredients starting with arugula. Set the jars in the refrigerator to cool.

2. Whisk all the items for dressing.

3. Put the dressing on top of the salads.

4. Shake the jars before eating.

6) LEMON RASPBERRY MOUSSE PIE:

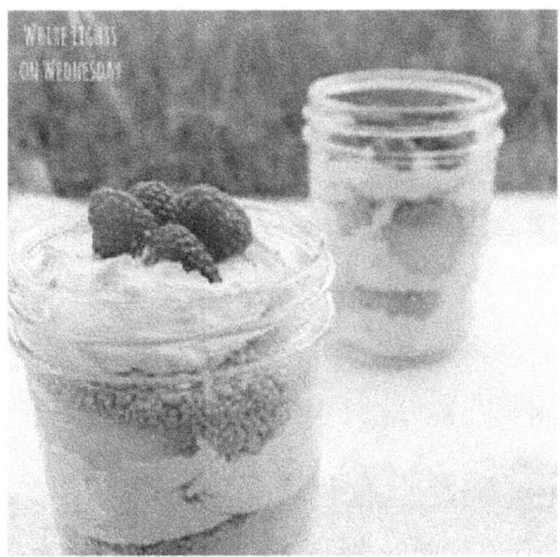

https://img.buzzfeed.com/buzzfeed-static/static/2014-07/7/19/enhanced/web-dr06/grid-cell-396-1404774781-3.jpg

This is an excellent prepping recipe for summers. Let's take a look at the ingredients,

- Thawed Vanilla Cool Whip Topping, (1 tub)

- Lucky Leaf Red Raspberry Pie Filling (3/4 cup)

- Lucky Leaf Lemon Pie Filling (1/2 cup)

- Graham cracker crumbs (1 cup)

- Melted unsalted butter (2 tbsp.)

- Fresh raspberries (if you like)

What to do?

1. Take small bowl and mix Graham cracker crumbs and butter. Mix it really well.

2. Take a medium bowl, mix and fold thawed Cool Whip and red raspberry pie filling in it. Combine it well and then keep it a aside.

3. Take mason jars and put 2 tbsp. of graham cracker crumbs in the bottom. Put 1/2 cup raspberry mousse on it. Then top it with 2 tbsp. of lemon pie filling. Repeat all the steps.

4. Add raspberries on top.

7) ANTIPASTO SALAD IN A JAR:

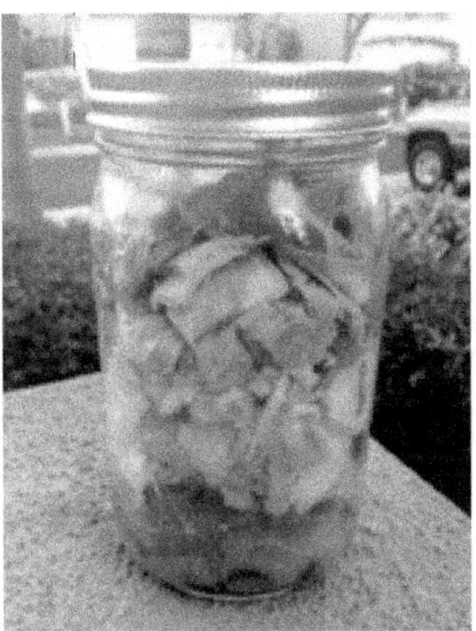

http://www.chaosandlove.com/wp-content/uploads/
2012/10/20121002-083712.jpg

This is a simple summer salad that is perfect for lunch. It's super fast. It would take only 20 minutes. Here are the ingredients,

- Salami, mortadella and capicola

- 1 head iceberg lettuce

- 4 Roma tomatoes

- Sliced pepperoncini (¼ cup)

- Sliced black olives (¼ cup)

- Olive oil (½ cup)

- Red wine vinegar (¼ cup)

- Salt and pepper

What to do?

1. Take a bowl and put oil, vinegar, salt and pepper in it and mix well.

2. Put tomatoes, pepperoncini and olives in it.

3. Take the meat and cut it in small pieces and put in the bowl with the mixture.

4. Fill the mason jars with this mixture.

5. Put lettuce on top.

6. Refrigerate the jars until you want to eat it.

8) STRAWBERRY AND GOAT CHEESE MASON JAR SALAD:

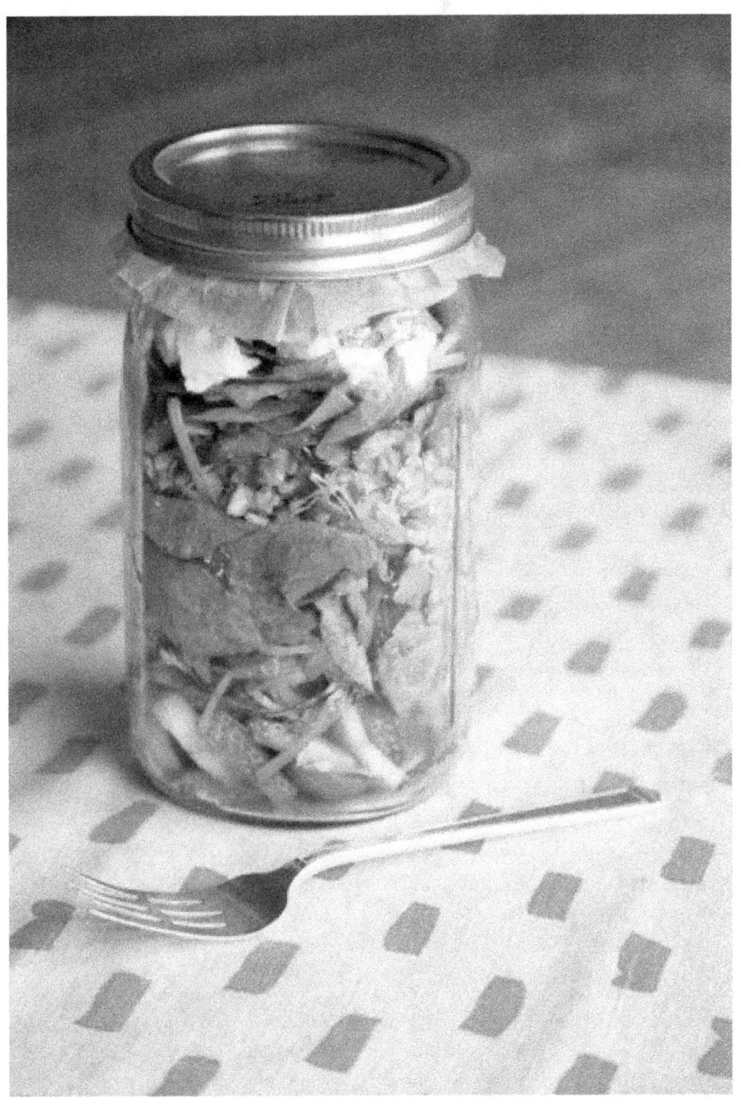

http://www.wellandgoodnyc.com/wp-content/uploads/2014/06/Strawberry-and-Goat-Cheese-Mason-Jar-Salad.jpg

This recipe is really simple and really very yummy. This salad includes the following ingredients,

- Sliced strawberries (2/3 cup)

- Spinach leaves (3 cups)

- Chopped walnuts (3 cups)

- Crumbled goat cheese (1.5 ounces)

- Balsamic vinaigrette or blueberry vinaigrette (2-3 tbsp.)

What to do?

1. Take a mason jar and put strawberries in the bottom. Next put salad dressing. Spinach comes next and then walnuts. Add the remaining spinach and put goat cheese on the top.

2. Put the vinaigrette and then seal the jar. Refrigerate the salad.

9) FRUIT & YOGURT BREAKFAST PARFAITS:

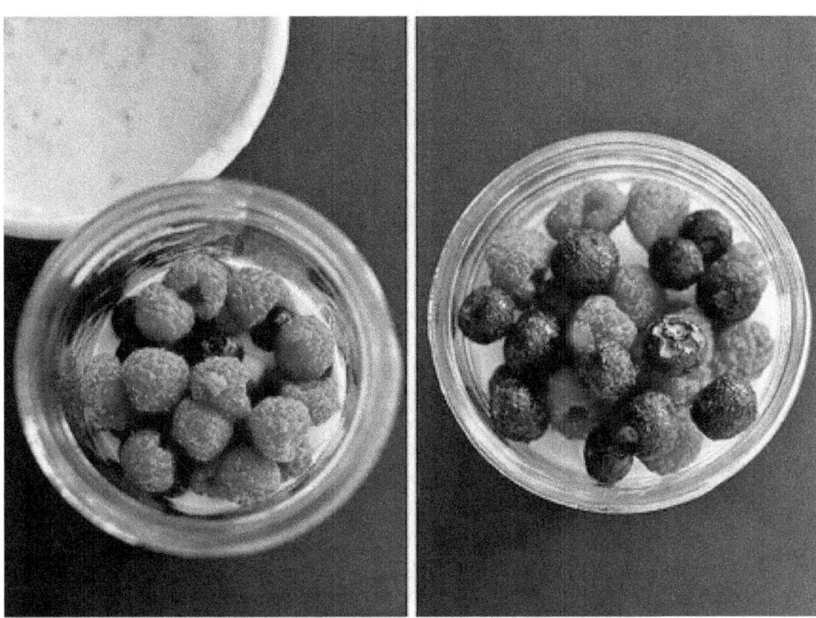

http://iowagirleats.com/2013/01/15/make-ahead-fruit-yogurt-breakfast-par-faits/makeaheadfruitandyogurtbreakfastparfaits_11_mini/

This is the perfect prepping recipe to cheer you up. Let's take a look at the ingre-dients,

- Uncooked certified gluten-free old fashioned oats (1/3 cup)

- Greek yogurt (6oz)

- Chia seeds (1 tsp)

- Milk (almond, cow, soy, etc.) (1 tbsp.)

- Frozen mixed fruit and berries (1 cup)

What to do?

1. Take a bowl and mix yogurt, oats, chia seeds, and milk in it.

2. Put a layer in Mason jar.

3. Add fruits and berries. Pour the remaining yogurt on top.

4. Garnish with berries.

5. Refrigerate until you're ready to eat.

10) CHICKPEA SALAD:

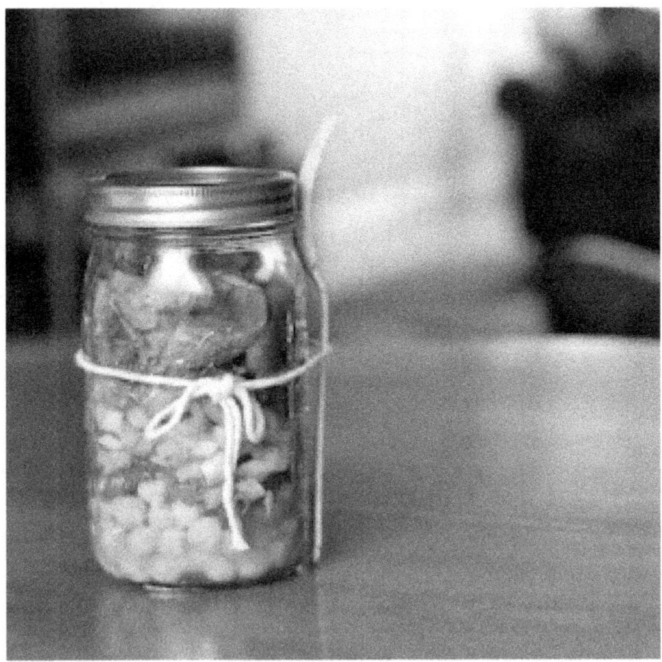

https://d3rgj9au57pk8c.cloudfront.net/uploaded/attachments/10803.jpg?v=befba6

This is another really simple salad that you can make in no time. A delight for you in summers. The items you need are,

- 2 tbsp. easy lemon vinaigrette (see below)

- Chickpeas (1 cup)

- sun-dried or oven roasted tomatoes (1/2 cup)

- Chopped Spring onion (1/4 cup)

- Chopped red onion (1/4 cup)

- Chopped olives (1/2 cup)

- Chopped piquillo peppers (1/4 cup)

- Fresh spinach (1/2 cup)

What to do?

Mix all the ingredients in a mason jar and refrigerate it until you're ready to eat.

Chapter 4 – What Food You Should Take During Prepping?

In this chapter, I would tell you what food you should keep and store during prepping. You don't want to miss anything that could be very healthy for you when you need it during unfavorable circumstances.

What food items should you store for prepping?

Now this is a hard decision because there are just so many things that you would to store. So make it easy for you, I'll ask you to store everything that you can. Not easy? It is if you have a list of everything you should store to help you survive when the circumstances take a very bad turn and you have to fight a surviving battle. Let's have a look at the list of everything that you should store for prepping,

Distilled water

Water is the most important thing that you'd need to survive in unfavorable conditions. You won't be able to make it for more than 3 days without water. So let's keep water on the top of the list of everything that you need to store. Make sure you've store plenty of water that is clean and pure.

Dehydrated powdered milk

Make sure you've bought enough powdered milk to keep in your storage.

Frozen dried eggs and powdered eggs

Buy frozen dried eggs and powdered eggs to keep in your storage. These eggs are 100% pure with no preservatives. Eggs usually last longer and don't need refrigeration.

Hard Cheese

To keep the cheese from rotting and catching bacteria, keep it stored in wax cases. This would keep the cheese from catching moisture too.

Protein bars and drinks

High in protein, protein bars and drinks are a must for your storage for they are a source of instant protein to your body.

Canned meat (Poultry, beef, mutton & seafood)

Meat is very important for human body. 90% of the sustenance required to survive is provided by meat. So make sure you save a lot of meat.

Coffee & tea

When you have to survive, it's essential that you stay alert. And for this you have to stock a lot of coffee and tea.

Essential cooking oils

To cook food, you'd need a lot oil. Make sure you stock a lot of oils in your storage. Stock olive oil, coconut oil, ghee, butter, lard and other essential oils.

Whole wheat flour

Stock a lot of wheat flour in your storage. A lot. Because you'll be needing wheat flour in a lot of your dishes.

1. Cereals, rice, corn etc.

2. Cornmeal, oats and oatmeal

3. Bread, crackers, pastas etc.

4. Jams and Jellies

5. Nuts, raisins, seeds etc.

6. Iodized salt

7. Sugar

8. Herbs and spices

9. Canned fruits and vegetables

10. Honey

11. Different sauces, vinegar

Make sure you get everything in enough quantities to keep in your storage room
for prepping. If you feel like adding some other things that you want in this list,
go on and do that.

Conclusion

One thing that is to be kept in mind when you prep is that you should not solely focus on food. Make sure you have other things with you too. You should have different medications, first-aid kits, enough amount of water to drink and to use for other purposes. Make sure you have everything you could need when the times are tough and adverse.

The recipes given in this book look fancy and flashy but they are really simple and really useful. You would not feel the severity of the circumstances if you are able to master some of these prepping recipes. You don't want to be thinking about how adverse the circumstances are, all the time. These recipes would not only help you feel better but they are really nutritious too.

You can either make your survival even tougher for you by eating food that is not tasty because you're too busy thinking about survival while you make your food. Or you can go ahead try these recipes that could help you lighten your mood even when you know times are hard. You have to positive. And to be positive, you would have to eat positive. Without being positive, you will not be able to survive as it is an essential thing to do. Best of luck!

Disappear Without A Trace

Introduction: Just Another Day... Just Another Footprint

For most of us, as we go about our day browsing the web or swiping our credit cards at stores for purchases, we don't give it much of a second thought. We hardly stop to think of the digital profile that all of these activities are creating. In the grand scheme of things there are two main categories when it comes to the digital footprints that we leave behind. And these two main categories are "active digital footprints" and "passive digital footprints".

When thinking of active digital footprints, think of your Face Book page, because these are online digital billboards where we are actively advertising intimate details of our lives. You post it and the whole world knows about it; pretty simple right? But when it comes to the passive digital footprint that we leave behind without even knowing it—things get considerably more complicated.

This is due to the fact that our passive digital footprints can be stored in an infinitely vast assortment of online environs. To show you just how easy it is to build up your passive digital database, just take a moment to consider all of the links and web pages that you absentmindedly click on any given day. No matter where you are, no matter what device you are using as an interface, every time you make that click, you are dropping off snippets of your passive digital footprint.

Each individual click is known as a "hit" which can be used to track the users IP address, right along with when the site was visited and even what type of computer and internet platform was used to access the site. Active digital footprints need to be managed, minimized, and if you so desire erased completely from public knowledge. In the modern world of rampant identity theft, protecting our most personal of data has become a full time responsibility.

But it's not just your digital footprint you have to worry about either; you also have to be cognizant of your offline tracks as well. Because no matter what you are doing you can't be complacent, in order to truly become invisible you have to be vigilant and practice it every single day of your life. Potential threats to your security can come from anywhere.

I'm not trying to spread fear and paranoia by telling you this, but the fact remains, we live in a very unpredictable world. Everything could be just fine one day and then your whole world could be turned upside down the next. In order to protect yourself as much as possible you have to take hold of your own identity and any corresponding information that comes with it.

You need to be able to control all information that leaves your possession, and whether that means shredding your paper documents before they hit the trashcan or using a P.O. Box to keep your address confidential, all of these things need to be maintained on a daily basis; because in the end its just another day and just another footprint you want to avoid.

Chapter 1: Eliminating your Active Digital Footprint

As was touched upon in the introduction of this book, most of us are actively creating our own digital footprint every single day. It could be as simple as posting a video on You Tube or adding a post to Face Book. The possibility for unique expression today is virtually endless, and as we will see in this chapter so are the consequences.

Facebook

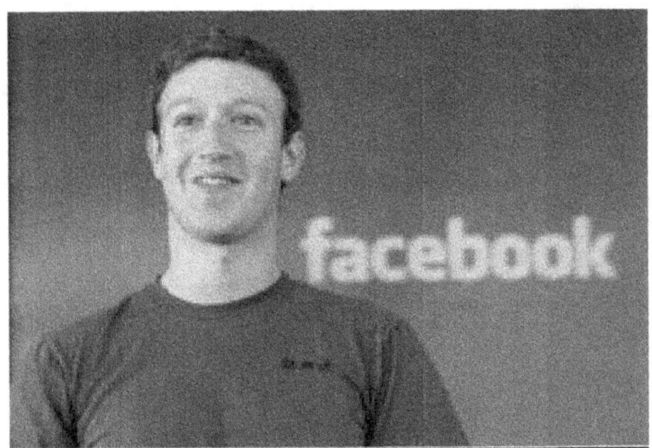

Ever since Mark Zuckerberg broke up with his girlfriend and decided to create a social network for hopeless geeks like himself we have all been at the mercy of this vast digital footprint collector! I am of course being somewhat facetious here but Face Book really is one of the most comprehensive online digital profiles ever conceived of. It is purposefully addictive in nature and pulls more and more information from its users every day they use the platform. It is practically unavoidable.

Even if you are not blatantly posting your address, phone number, and birthday, if you have an active Face Book account there are still no doubt a wide variety of minor details that can be collected about you to form a basic digital footprint. If you wish to minimize the impact of a social media platform like this, always set your Face Book page to private, this will at least prevent you from creating an active digital footprint.

But in the end if you really wish to eliminate your active digital footprint you will need to delete all of your Face Book accounts. Because Face Book itself is a security risk, leaking information on a daily basis, it needs to be controlled. Having that said, the best lesson I could give to someone who is wanting to disappear without a trace. If you have Face Book; get rid of it.

Linkedin

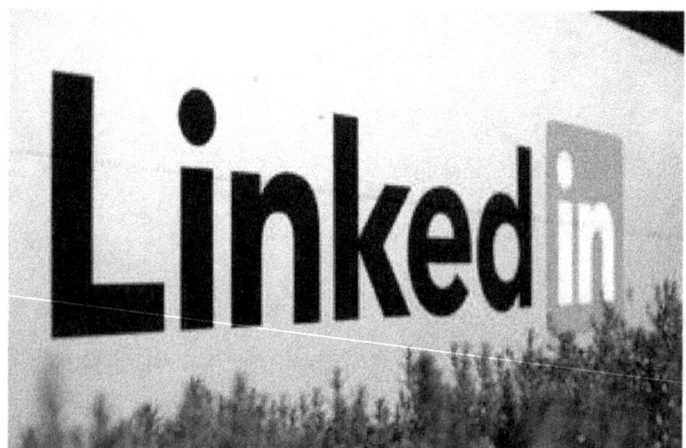

Although Linkedin is supposed to be the premiere site when it comes to meeting professionals and landing the right job, it is also a way to create an immense digital footprint of data that can last for decades. And as it turns out Linkedin is also prime hunting ground for hackers. Because if someone could get a hold of the virtual resume you post on Linkedin they have a veritable treasure trove of information.

Just look at what happened in 2012 when one hacker compromised 6.5 million passwords of registered Linkedin users. These hacks were then followed up by phishing schemes designed to gather even more information from the targets. If you would like to disappear, Linkedin could cause you a major problem. So if you would like to cut down on your digital information you would definitely need to consider getting rid of your Linkedin.

You Tube

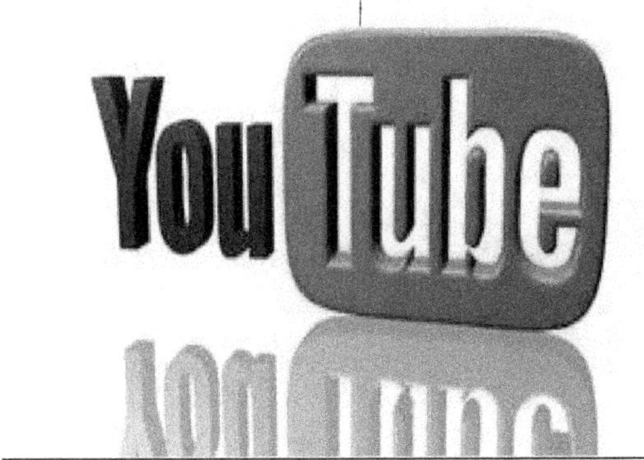

We all love You Tube, we love watching all of the cat video's, music performances, and epic fails that fill our computer. But as entertaining as these things are, our purveyance of them leaves a very unique algorithm in its wake. And much more than this if you have an account and post your own videos through the service you are becoming an active advertising partner. It's not all gloom and doom however, because if you are trying to disappear without a trace it is feasible to use You Tube as a bit of a smoke screen.

You can do this by deliberately posting videos and profile information that has nothing at all to do with you and who you are and then abruptly stop your activity with that account. This could potentially work as diversion for anyone that might be on your trail. So that is my ultimate lesson for you when it comes to You Tube either use it as a disinformation channel for your whereabouts or delete your You Tube account.

Twitter

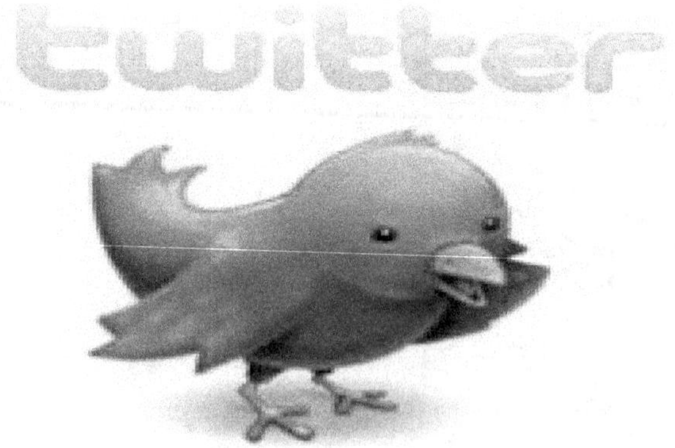

Ah, twitter; the mouthpiece of the world and best friend of Donald Trump! But as much as we enjoy it, whether you are a Presidential candidate or just a regular Joe Schmo down the block, Twitter could be the single most devastating platform when it comes to trying to minimize a digital footprint. Because twitter is like a megaphone announcing to the world your innermost thoughts, and as we have seen during this heated election season, this can be a good thing and a very bad thing!

And one of the toughest things about twitter is that even if you delete posts or even delete your account, anyone who liked your tweets can carry them on for you indefinitely. This can be particularly devastating if your account gets hacked into. I had a friend once who lost control of his account and had someone post ridiculous statements under his name. It took him ages to clear up all the awful things that he never even said!

So let this be a lesson to you; twitter can make and break you. Twitter works as an instantaneous platform to express your own unique persona and if someone were to control this powerful means of expression they will control you. So just to be on the safe side, if you would like to disappear you are going to have to break that twitter habit.

Word press

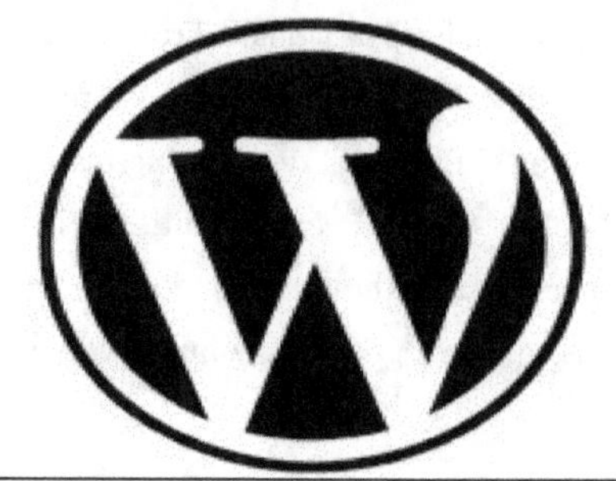

Word press is great for bloggers and budding writers alike. Being a writer myself, I have lent a few of my own masterpieces to this free writing platform. But all of those opinionated blogs and articles that you cram into word press have a way of sneaking back up on you. They are not going to go anywhere anytime soon, so yes, if you would like to disappear you will have to avoid word press too.

Chapter 2: Eliminating your Passive Digital Footprint

As mentioned in the previous chapter there is a great deal of online activity that we voluntarily contribute to our digital footprint and presence online. But as much as we do things intentionally to build up a digital profile there are many other things that we make constant contributions to that we are blithely unaware of. Because unbeknownst to us there are whole data collecting agencies out there stockpiling all of your absent minded clicks, comments and browsing habits. In this chapter we are going to take a look at some of the most common ways that your passive digital footprints are being created.

Google

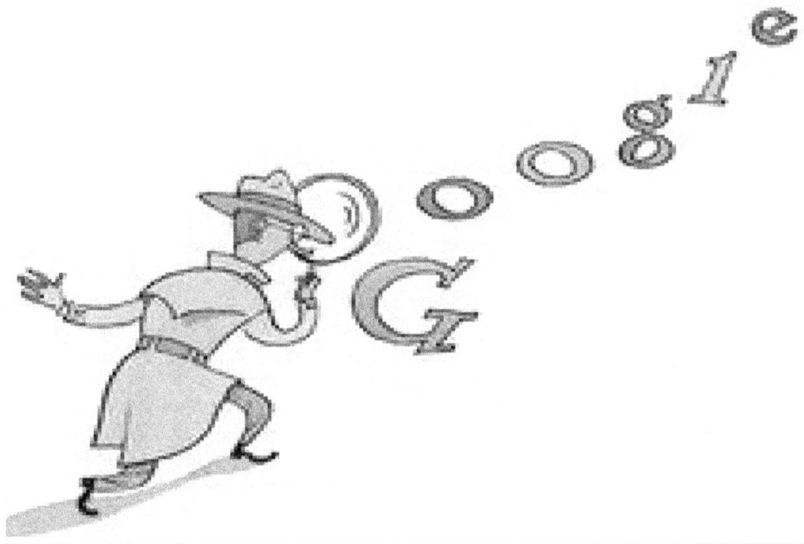

Google is an amazing beast of information and we use it so much that the name has become a part of the lexicon. Surely you have "Googled" something right? The problem is that we all have. And all of this googling by everyone you know has created quite a mountain of information, likes, dislikes and preferences. Like all search engines, Google uses cookies to track where you go while you are on the internet.

These sneaky little cookies gather up all of your personal details so that advertisers can have effective strategies to market products to you based on your online habits. But it isn't only the folks that want to sell you things that keep track of this data. Because there are whole companies known as "Data Gatherers" that store up all the information they can glean from Google and then turn around and sell that info for a price.

From just a thorough scouring of your internet cookies these guys manage to deduce your name, address, age, phone number, previous addresses, occupations and even hobbies. With this passive digital footprint they can follow a trail of cookies all the way back to you. In order to disappear from this digital dragnet you should always optimize your web browser to refuse all cookies.

And not only are the guys at Google busy shaping up these intense digital profiles based upon your clicks and cookies, now because Google is somehow linked to most people's e-mails they are also directly getting information about you through your email account. It is not quite understood why Google wants you to log in with your e-mail in order to search for information on burrito's (or whatever else you are looking up) but it seems to prefer if you are.

The lesson to be learned here is that Google is fast becoming one of the number one data collecting sights on the internet. And so if you really want to disappear you are better off not having this one as a part of your online repertoire. So yes, get rid of Google if you would like to eliminate your passive digital footprint.

Amazon

Amazon is the most popular marketplace on the planet right now and they sell just about everything that you could ever imagine, but did you know that they sell your information as well? Every time you buy something or even just browse through the description of a product Amazon takes note and saves your chosen preferences for a later date. The details of your purchase can be saved for years. Big deal right?

Well—although this may seem rather arbitrary on the surface, these details add up, and can lead to quite an extensive digital footprint. Amazon captures your browsing details by enticing you not only to buy but to comment and rate other products as well. You may think that you are just informing others of how great that last book you read on Amazon was, but you're really just telling them a lot of unnecessary information about yourself. In order to make your online profile vanish, stay away from Amazon.

Ask

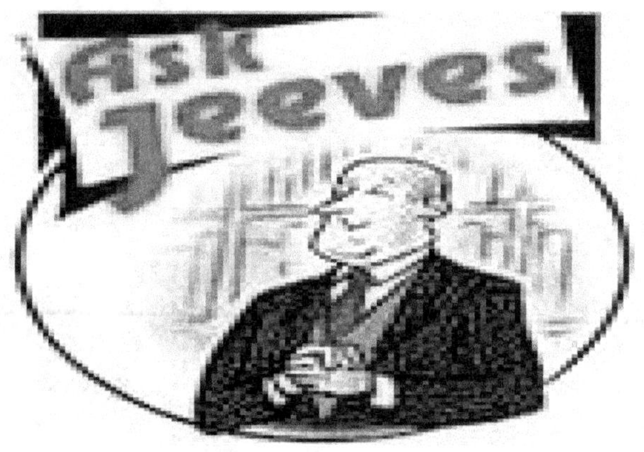

I used to love ask.com. I even remember the good old days when it was known as AskJeeves.com. I loved to see that happy little butler answering all of my questions, and allaying all of my hopes and fears. But I hate to break it to you folks, but that self same company that brought you that chipper butler also took all of your information. Many people have complained about the Ask toolbar that seems to install itself after too many browsing sessions.

This toolbar is unwanted adware at its best and harmful malware at its worst. This software has often been inserted into unsuspecting users computers by bundling together with Java updates. Once installed this toolbar tracks practically everything you do on your computer, storing all of the passive footprints you make for later use. And just like any insidious parasite, the toolbar is not easy to remove. It will fight you all the way, often causing serious system crashes and disruptions just from attempting to delete the program.

To show you just how sneaky the guys over at Ask were when they created this toolbar, they designed it with a delay feature, so that it lays dormant (like a virus maybe?) in your computer and does not present itself immediately after you (accidentally) install it. This toolbar will then show up out of nowhere days later to start sucking up all of your data like a massive cyber leach. So if anything else, in order to avoid this horrible fate, if you are trying to disappear, stay as far away from "Ask" as you possibly can.

E-mail

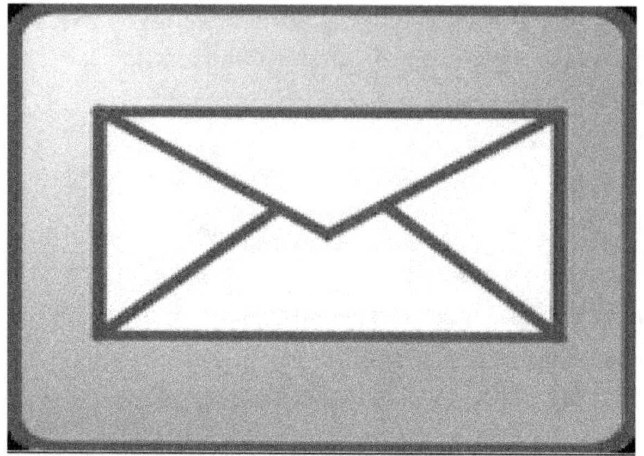

This lesson in disappearing without a trace is a rather general one, because we all have e-mail. And for most of us, checking our email is as much of a part of our routine as brushing our teeth. But all of this mindless e-mail checking creates quite a trail of passive digital footprints for anyone who might be paying attention, because a simply search of our e-mail log will tell someone where we are when we checked our email, what time of day that we checked and for how long of a duration.

Seemingly simple tidbits of information but when you wish to disappear they can become quite burdensome. The other problem with e-mails is that they can be too easily hacked into. So easy, that even Presidential candidate's such as Hillary Clinton have been hacked. This is because many of us have passwords that are just way too easily guessed. A recent survey found that the most popular passwords for e-mails are 123456, 12345, password, and qwerty.

As you can see none of these are the least bit imaginative, with two of them being just a series of numbers counting forward, one being literally the word "password" and the brilliant "Querty" simply being how the first 5 letters appear on a keyboard, these simplistic passphrases are checked every single day by any resourceful hacker. Even if they don't just guess the generic passwords off the top of their heads, the second they run a hacking oriented computer program all bets are off because that software will skim easy passwords like these right off the top of the list.

And once someone has access to your e-mail they can just about unravel your entire identity, so if you are going to have an e-mail address make sure that it is incredibly complex using a combination of letters, numbers and symbols, and only use it sparingly otherwise you could be compromised. The best way to disappear however is to not have an e-mail address at all. Having that said, I can say that I sympathize completely with Bernie Sanders when he expressed, "I'm sick and tired of hearing about your damn e-mails!"

MapQuest

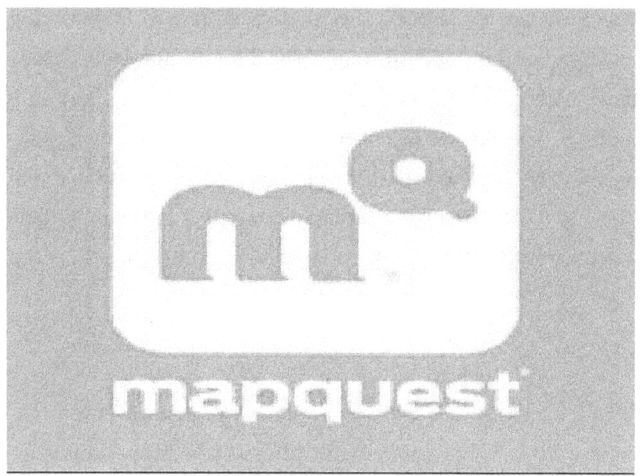

How many times have we used MapQuest in order to plot our locations when we are lost on some misadventure road trip? In a matter of seconds after plotting in the coordinates you can generate some pretty accurate directions. The only trouble is; directions are not the only thing that MapQuest generates because it also tracks your location and not only that, it stores all of those trips you've ever plotted, leaving all of them stored in the MapQuest database for an indefinite period of time.

Did you enjoy all of those summer trips to Florida? Well guess what? MapQuest enjoyed it too! It enjoyed tracking your whereabouts and traveling preferences during your entire sojourn in the Sunshine State! MapQuest knows exactly where you went because you told them all about it! So if you wish to truly disappear your best bet is to use an old fashioned paper road map!

Chapter 3: Burner Phones, P.O. Boxes and Gerbils Oh My!

So far in this book we have discussed cyber security and how to minimize the shadow that our online habits may create. Now let's take the time to think about all of our offline activities that would need to be minimized and brought under strict monitoring in order to truly disappear from the radar.

Because despite the complexities of today's world, there are still many things you can do to curtail your presence. The main thing to come to grips with is that you are the gatekeeper to your own identity and what it is that gets leaked out. Learn how to control this flow of information and you can control who can see you and who can not.

Cell Phones

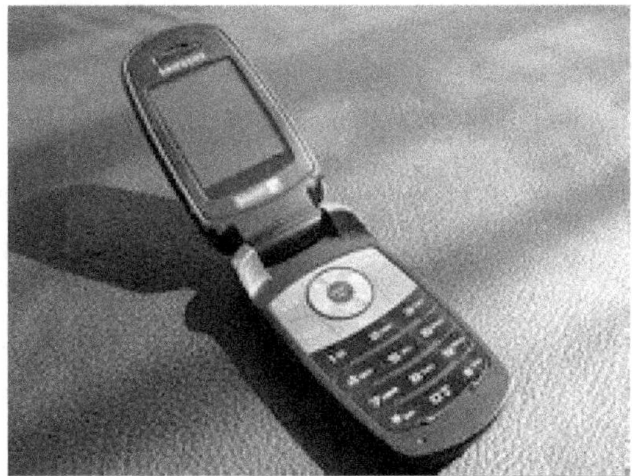

We all love our cell phones, but little do we know that these little gadgets that we all have stuffed right in pockets, purses, and who knows where else are GPS tracking devices. That's right, as long as that phone is turned on, anyone who cares to look into it can find your physical location. Because when your phone is turned on it sends out a constant signal to the nearest cell phone tower, which then gives whoever may be paying attention a pretty good idea of where you are at all times.

So as a rule, if you do use a cell phone, you should turn it off as soon as you are done using it, so you aren't sending out a constant beacon informing others of your whereabouts. This is why having reliable voicemail is important, so you can leave the phone off and then just periodically check it for messages. Only using a phone for when you really need it and turning it off when its not in use is also very conducive for a pay as you go phone or as they are euphemistically referred to "burner phones".

They are named as such because you can basically burn right through these phones and then throw them away. These phones can be used by anyone with none of your personal information attached to it. There is no contract, no deposit, no credit check and no identification required to activate one of these phones. All you have to do is pick one up from Wal-Mart (or wherever you get it from) and pay for the phone and any phone card to supply minutes to the device, all in cash. Follow this lesson and it will be much easier for you to completely disappear when you need to.

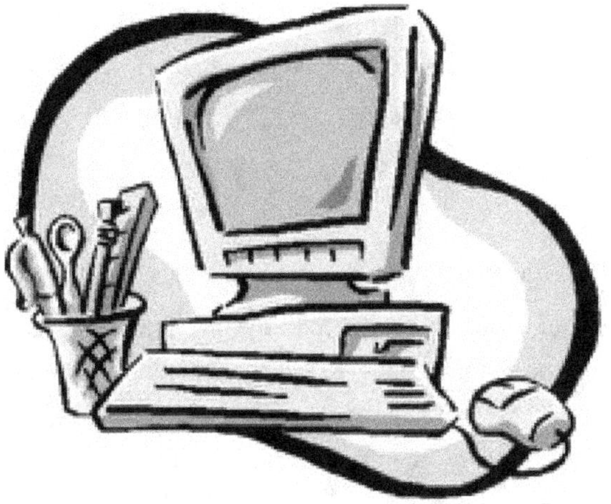

We have been living in the so-called "computer age" for the past 30 years now and you will be hard pressed to found a home anywhere without at least one computing device. Through the internet computer activity can permeate everything we do and we have already touched upon some of the dangers entailed when it comes to online privacy and security. But what you may not realize about computers is that even when they are not connected to the internet they could pose a danger to your personal information.

If anyone breaks into your house and steals your laptop for example, despite the fact that you may have never even took that computer online, your information is now in the hands of thieves. And believe it or not, even without someone physically breaking into your home or hacking into your database through the internet there are still other means by which someone can still your information right off of your computer.

Amazingly if someone had the equipment, they could park a car down the block from your house and pick up your "Van Eck" emissions. This is the steady signal that your computer monitor leaks out and from this signal just about anyone can piece together every single thing on your screen even when you are offline. Sounds pretty scary doesn't it?

Well, as frightening as it is, the only real way to solve these potential breaches in security is to load up our computer with encrypted files. By encrypting your files you are basically jumbling up the main components of the data and recording them in an indecipherable code so that if prying eyes are trying to steal your info they will have a hard time understanding the information that they have lifted. You should also consider creating what is known as "multiple rings" of security or defense.

The first layer of defense for your computer is to make sure that the data contained within it is mobile and can be carried with you when you if need be. The easiest way to achieve this is to use laptops and notebooks; otherwise you should make sure that the hard drive in your desktop is easy to pull out, so you can simply take the hard drive with you when you leave. The next layer of your computer security should be securing the room in which you work with your computer.

All of these precautions may seem rather intense, but as we have seen in this book, if you really want to make 100% sure that know one can compromise your data then you need to really go out on a limb and make that extra effort. So having that said, the first step towards making your room a safe zone free from possible infiltration is to keep the computer away from windows, this is to eliminate the chance of surveillance equipment being used to target your computer. Also if you can try to put a steel plate up on the other side of your door or some other kind of reinforcement to block any radiation or signals that might be leaking from your device.

The next way to safeguard your computer is to use multiple hard drives. You should take two hard drives and install the same operating system on each drive. When you are working with sensitive data you should use the same drive for that purpose, and then when you are done you can ten revert back to the identical drive and take the confidential one out with you when you leave. That way if anyone ever stole your computer you wouldn't lose anything important. These few security measures make it a whole lot easier if you need to disappear.

Use A Gerbil as a Living Shredder

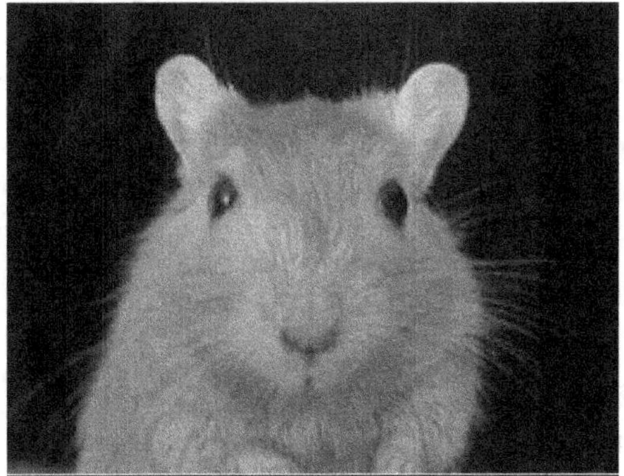

I admit this one sounds awfully strange. And you may have laughed when you saw this heading, but using a Gerbil to shred documents is one of the most effective and efficient means I have discovered when it come to getting rid of sensitive documents. If you have ever had a Gerbil (You know those furry little guys you get from the pet store that look kind of like a cuter version of the rat?) you probably know what I'm talking about though. Because these guys love to shred paper!

They are constantly chewing on stuff and when you hand them strips of paper, they will shred it down into tiny bits and pieces with the consistency of confetti. What I usually do is I take my documents and I shred them through a normal mechanical shredder into conventional strips of shredded paper. But then instead of tossing these shreds into the trash where if someone wanted to they could simply piece them back together again—instead of doing that—I drop the strips right into my Gerbil's cage and he starts working on those pieces of paper immediately.

He's an expert—I've timed the little guy before and he seems to average about one paper strip every 30 seconds. So you give him 8 strips of mechanically shredded paper from one document and he will have all eight of those strips converted into unrecognizable bits and pieces within about 4 minutes. The Gerbil loves this stuff and he will use this now confetti-like paper as his bedding—tunneling in it, sleeping in it, rolling around in it, and yes, even pooping and peeing in it until there is no possible way that anyone could ever glean any possible data from those shredded docs ever again.

I hope you aren't thoroughly disgusted by the concept, but a paper loving animal like a Gerbil can completely annihilate your sensitive documents faster than any mechanical shredder ever could. So yes, for this lesson I seriously suggest investing in a Gerbil just so it can shred all of your documents. Because if you want to disappear and lose your paper trail, a Gerbil's incredible shredding ability is a natural aid in this process.

Post Office Box

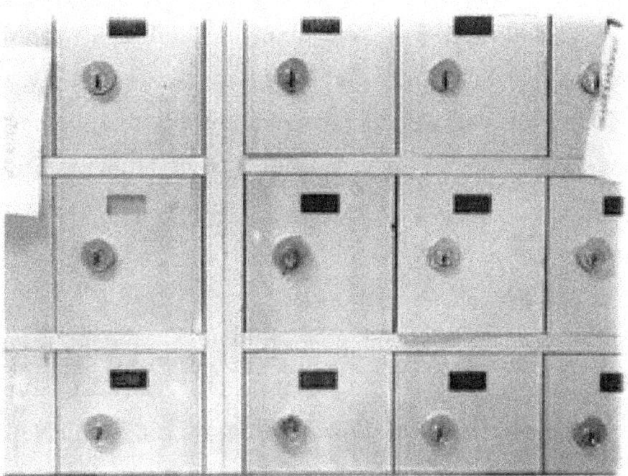

In the information age we think quite a bit about securing our digital information such as e-mails, but we would be very silly to secure our cyber correspondence but then not give any thought whatsoever to our physical mail in the mail box. Because whether you live in an apartment or a house you most likely get flooded with little paper pieces of information everyday and some of it is extremely revealing about your personal assets and situation.

All of this can be solved however by shutting down your fixed mailbox and redirecting all of your physical correspondence to an old fashioned Post Office Box. The best way to go about doing this is to rent out a private mailbox that is issued by a commercial mail group and then list the P.O. Box under a company name, designating it for magazine subscriptions, or business correspondence.

At the time of opening this P.O. Box your current physical street address is no doubt all over the place, so in order to help that piece of the puzzle disappear, when you move to a new address, do not give it out to anyone and then turn to the P.O. Box that you have already established for all future correspondence. The P.O. Box is not only more secure for your personal information it is also a means to shield your actual street address from prying eyes helping your actual physical location disappear from the radar.

And here's one more tip for helping you shake the paper trail of your old address; get a P.O. Box that is as far away from your starting location as you can. Now I'm not talking about going crazy and renting a P.O. Box in Chicago if you live in New York, but try not to get a P.O. that's in a 5 mile radius of your starting locale. Try to get a P.O. that puts a little bit of distance between you and your starting spot but yet is still convenient enough for you to check at least once a weak.

Limited Liability Company

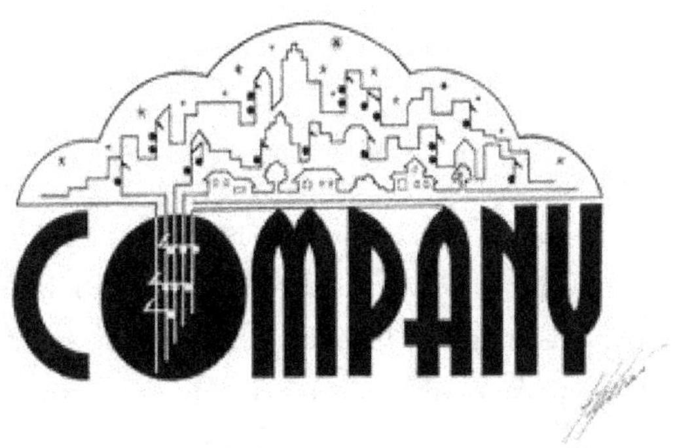

LLC? Surely you have seen this arrangement of these three letters on countless business cards, addresses and solicitation. But what exactly is a Limited Liability Company? Just as the name implies it is a legal entity with very limited liability meaning that no one knows who the owner is unless the owner expressly tells them and it is managed by one single person who lists their LLC as a business address. Obtaining an LLC costs less than $100 and with this you can register cars and license plates under this heading helping you to disappear from unwanted scrutiny.

Conclusion: A Lifetime of Management

We live in a world of constant surveillance. If it's not our online traffic being monitored then it is our physical every day traffic on the streets being scrutinized by thousands of security cameras. Everything in today's world is tracked and compartmentalized inside some database somewhere. So how is it in such a world of scrutiny we could ever hope of holding on to any sense of privacy or security? By common sense and the detailed management of our lives, and I hope that this book has provided you with the tools you need to do just that.

Home Defense

Introduction

To begin with, this book includes in itself a detailed analysis about how to secure your home from external dangers. In order to answer this question, this book includes various perspectives about how to eradicate this threat and secure your house. Therefore, this book expound upon some of the tips and techniques that ensure safety.

Firstly, planning the basic security is the most essential thing to provide safety. Therefore, this book includes certain techniques about basic security planning. Secondly, physical defense is among the most important techniques that can help you secure yourself from all types of threats. Thus, a guide is provided regarding how to learn this technique. Moreover, the importance of physical defense is also elaborated. Thirdly, all of the essential armories to secure your house are also discussed in detail. Fourthly, tips about keeping guard dogs are involved to help the reader in training these types of dogs. In the end, another important aspect i.e. techniques to secure the children and disabled people is also added in the coming text.

Therefore, this constellation of techniques for security of your beloved home and family is a book worth-reading. It not only serves as a manual for home security but also it includes in self the details about the importance of these techniques. In addition to that, the precautionary measures that must be adopted by the individuals are also another amazing aspect of this book. Thus, this book enables a person to learn the techniques required for a secure home.

Chapter 1 – Basic Security Planning

You might have been blessed with safe neighborhood, yet heinous activities happen all around. Therefore, it is essential to secure your relatives and individual property against lawbreakers who may attempt to break into your house and hinder the safety of your family. Thus, in order to ensure everybody in your family, device a plan such that all members are well aware of the strategies to secure themselves from any mishap. The most ideal approach to keep everybody in the planning is by the creation of a security planning at home. Create a home security arrangement for your home by assembling an agenda of all that you have to do to keep your home sheltered and after that imparting that arrangement to your relatives.

Following is the things that must be considered while developing a security plan:

- **Create a financial plan:**

The home security arrangement must include the items you have bought along with the money spent on them. Moreover, the budget must have the amount you can spend on your home's security.

- **Check your windows and doors:**

1. Any security arrangement must incorporate in itself plans to hinder the entrance of intruders in your house using doors and windows.

2.   Ensure that the windows and doors are kept bolted. Moreover, these locks must be created using high quality material. For instance, your outside entryways must not be weak enough to be easily broken

3.   Introduce strike plates efficiently. This is the metal plate that is joined to your door frame. It will keep the lock and bolt secure

4.   Check the hinges of your windows and doors. They must be installed in a secure manner. However, if your door has a window on it then it must be in a good shape and not in a need of substitution

- **Take care of any wall or doors you have on your property:**

On the off chance that there are openings or harms to your wall or door, plan to have them repaired or supplanted.

- **Introduce walls or doors:**

Consider introducing a wall or a door on the off chance that you do not possess one right now. They can help you keep individuals and creatures off your property.

- **Security gadgets:**

Figure out what security gadgets you have, and which you might require. You might need a basic deadbolt or a simple alarm system attached to each of the window and door. Moreover, numerous individuals build their home security by introducing cameras, alarm catches and sensors on their property.

- **Security signs:**

Post signs which depict that your house is observed 24 hours a day. Then again, consider a sign that cautions individuals drawing closer of alarms and guard dogs.

- **Illuminate your house:**

1. Make lighting a piece of your home security arrangement. All of the exterior regions near your home must be illuminated.

2. Indoor lighting is fundamental as well. A couple of lights ought to be left on in the home if you are out of your house.

- **Incorporate an emergency arrangement:**

(1) Your home security arrangement ought to contain guidelines to all relatives on what to do and where to go if something bad happen at home.

(2) Choose where you will meet if there is a crisis. This may be a neighbor's home, a relative's home or an open place that is anything but difficult to get to.

- **Keep your information hidden:**

Share the information just with individuals who need to know it. Try not to give out your home security code or leave your key outside in an undeniable area.

- Make an outline that will highlight all those area that are alarmed and also where you keep the pepper shower or other cautious apparatuses.

- Incorporate telephone quantities of your nearby police headquarters and in addition companions and relatives. Try not to let this arrangement outside of your home, or your security will be traded off.

Your security plan must fulfill following points:

-       Details of the defensive efforts to establish safety to be executed, covering physical, data and faculty security.

-       Guidelines on the methods for proficient reaction to a risk.

-       Tips to react on suspicious events

-       Evacuation arrangements including a detailed analysis on securing premises in case of a full clearing

-       An interchanges and media methodology which likewise incorporates taking care of inquiries from concerned family and companions.

Chapter 2 – Physical Defense Techniques

Would you have the capacity to shield yourself and your friends and family if somebody was to physically assault you? It's an inquiry the vast majority of us would prefer not to consider, however viciousness is, sadly, an unavoidable truth. Thankfully, paying little mind to quality, size, or past preparing, anybody can take in a few successful self-preservation procedures.

1.   **Push and yell:**

When the assailant touches you or even when the escape is impractical, shout noisily and push back at him or her. This does two things: it signals for help and it tells the aggressor you are not a simple target. It may not discourage all aggressors, but rather getting noisy will caution off those that were searching for simple prey.

2.   **Hurt the sensitive parts of attacker:**

When a person is in an encounter with an attacker, you just have a few moments and a couple moves to attempt before the attacker is done. Before, the aggressor has gained full control of you, you should do all that you can. So go for the parts of the body where you can do the most harm effectively:

i.   Eyes

ii.   Ears

iii.   Crotch

iv.   Legs

v.   Knees

vi.   Neck

Following depicts the ways to hit the critical areas:

Contingent upon the position of the assailant and how close he is will figure out where you will hit and which part of your body will you utilize. Try not to venture in closer, say, to hit his nose with your hand, when you can achieve his knee with a kick.

At the point when striking an objective on the upper portion of the body you will utilize your hand. Successful hits can be made with the external edge of your hand in a blade hand position, a palm strike or knuckle blow for milder targets or a firmly twisted clench hand.

Eyes:

Gouging, jabbing, or even scratching the assailant's eyes with your fingers or knuckles would be successful, as you can envision. Other than bringing on a lot of pain, this must also make your departure less demanding by at any rate incidentally meddling with his vision.

Nose:

If by chance the aggressor is close to you, utilize the heel of your palm to strike up under his nose; toss the entire weight of your body into the move to bring about the most torment and compel him to slacken his grasp on you. In the event that he's behind you, you can hit his nose with your elbow. In any case, go for the nasal bones.

Neck:

The side of the neck is a greater target, where both the carotid supply route and jugular vein are found. You could briefly paralyze your assailant with a blade hand strike-all fingers held straight and firmly together, with thumb tucked and somewhat bowed at the knuckle along the edge of the neck. For significantly more damage, you could push your elbow into your attacker's throat while pitching the heaviness of your body forward.

Knee:

Knee is a perfect self-preservation target, helpless from each point and effortlessly kicked without danger of your foot being gotten. Kick the side of the knee to bring about damage or in part cripple your aggressor. Kicking the front of the knee may bring about more harm however is less inclined to bring about lopsidedness.

For optimum damage:

In order to cause maximum damage to the attacker, following techniques can be beneficial:

- **Utilize your knees, elbows, and head:**

Those are the parts of the body that are most delicate when hit. Presently the parts of the body utilized most successfully to inflict harm are your elbows, head and knees.

-        **Use regular items:**

Ordinary items you bear with you or things in your surroundings can likewise be utilized further bolstering your good fortune as weapons. Hold a key or pen between your center and ring finger while you're strolling home oblivious for more affirmation. Outside, you can hurl some dirt or sand into your aggressor's eyes. Ladies are regularly advised to splash fragrance or hairspray into an aggressor's eyes.

-        **Balance your weight:**

Regardless of your size, weight, or quality in connection to your adversary, you can guard yourself by deliberately utilizing your body and the straightforward law of material science. This is the rule behind hand to hand fighting frameworks like Jujitsu and other self-protection programs where a littler individual can overcome a bigger one.

Helpful moves to fight attackers:

Following are some helpful techniques that can help you in fighting an attacker. These moves can further help you in escaping.

-        **Wrist Hold:**

Gracie Jiu-Jitsu is another school of self-preservation, one that offers changed Jujitsu systems that comparatively feeble individuals can complete. Rather than pulling back to attempt to escape the hold, hunch down into a solid position, then incline forward and twist your elbow towards him the distance towards his lower arm until he can no more clutch your wrist.

-       **Front and Back Choke Holds:**

This technique recommends twisting your elbow into escape the wrist hold, yet then pushing upwards to break free. The video additionally offers methods to escape a front strangle hold and a back strangle hold: Swing one arm crosswise over to break the assailant's hold then utilize your other arm's elbow or deliver a blade strike position to hit the aggressor.

-       **Mount Position:**

In case the assailant has you stuck on the floor, you can rotate to be on top with this Gracie Jiu-Jitsu method. Snare onto his wrist with one hand and utilize your other hand to get behind his elbow, catching his arm to your mid-section. At that point utilize your foot to trap his foot and leg, hips must be lifted and then turn your knees over so you can get on the top.

Chapter 3 – Essential Armory to Protect Your House

The normal robber or home intruder is searching for a simple target. For them wrongdoing is about danger versus reward. For the criminal the danger is getting gotten or shot. The prize is getting your resources, cash or you.

On the off chance that you, as the property holder, can up their danger they are more averse to pick your home. While burrowing a canal and encompassing your home with razor wire would absolutely make your home substantially more secure, it most likely would not run over genuine well with your neighbors.

So how would you make your home have all the earmarks of being a higher danger? How about we begin at the edge and work our way in.

1. Set up a fringe for your property. This builds up an unmistakable line of division. The fringe might be a wall, finishing or whatever else you may think of.

2. Show security alert signs in the front yard. The thought is the criminal will see the sign and proceed onward to a house that doesn't have security. Robbers can be in and out of a house in a matter of minutes yet late reports propose police in substantial urban communities will react in 30+ minutes on the off chance that they react by any stretch of the imagination.

3.   Trim the greenery to dispose of concealing spots, particularly around windows and entryways. That delightfully fragrant Gardenia Bush is flawless yet it may give the ideal concealing spot to a criminal. Adjusting your scene to incorporate thorny things may likewise demoralize robbers. Nothing entirely like experiencing a thistle bramble to deter one from one's planned way.

4.   Use lights in the night. Position the lights in a manner that dull spots are dispensed with. Movement finder lights are great, yet just actuate once movement is unique.

5.   Expel objects in the yard that could be utilized to help a cheat get to your home.

6.   Strengthen your windows with movies and equipment.

7.   The front entryway is the main section for home intruders and criminals. There are different strides you can take to improve the security of your front entryway.

8.   Substitute your screen entryway with an enriching iron security entryway and keep it bolted!

9.   Ensure your front entryway is strong. Empty center entryways are extremely feeble.

10.   Fortify the pivots with 3 inches screws, the door frame with strike plates, and ensure you have a decent dead fastener.

11.   Glass on or close to your entryway is likewise a frail spot in your security. I would recommend strengthening it with the same film as the windows.

12.   Introduce and utilize a peephole.

13.   Try not to open the way to outsiders. While this sounds straightforward, a huge segment of home intrusions happen when a tenant opens the entryway. As often as possible a home intruder will utilize an imitation to thump on your entryway. This individual might be a youngster offering magazines, a man wearing an utility uniform or a woman requesting that utilization the telephone since her auto separated.

These home defense plans for your family should be created, set, checked, tried, retested, and refined before it can be viable. At that point, the arrangement must be practiced and retained with the goal that it becomes receptive rather than thought-based. You don't have at whatever time to think when part second choices must be made. Or maybe, you should originate from a spot knowing instead of speculation in a crisis circumstance like a vicious assault or home attack.

When somebody breaks into your home, these plans must be ready to go constantly. There is no space for faltering. Your life and the welfare of your family are in your grasp. So this is the manner by which you get ready: Take the time now, right at the moment, to construct a reasonable home protection arrange and teach yourself on every one of the angles that you may feel you are deficient in.

Chapter 4 – Guard Dogs for Your House

All through history, one of the primary employments of the tamed puppy has been to secure its proprietors and make preparations for undesirable individuals or creatures. While numerous dogs will instinctively go about as home gatekeepers, there are particular breeds that are known for having the qualities expected to best avoid undesirable interlopers.

For quite a long time, dogs have been tamed; people have utilized them to monitor their domesticated animals and homes. Some breeds improve at comprehension one proprietor, and different breeds comprehend the whole family and will ensure every part just as it were one of its own. We have examined and positioned some of the best guard dogs for families, and have presented to you that rundown underneath. Ensure, as you look over this rundown, to keep on researching the breed you feel most nearly matches the needs of your family. This rundown is an extraordinary hopping of point for you and we feel every breed underneath brings a colossal measure of adoration and insurance to you your family.

1.   German shepherd:

German Shepherds, as we would see it, beat the rundown of best family protection dogs because of their normal senses to tune in, learn, and comply. They are both threatening in their appearance, and adoring in their temperament, yet will react to the call on any minutes notice. They have thick hide, which makes them react well to colder temperatures, and it adds to their sturdiness. They are extremely comprehension of their homes, and will be careful about gatecrashers.

They have phenomenal size and can bring down any estimated human without much inconvenience.

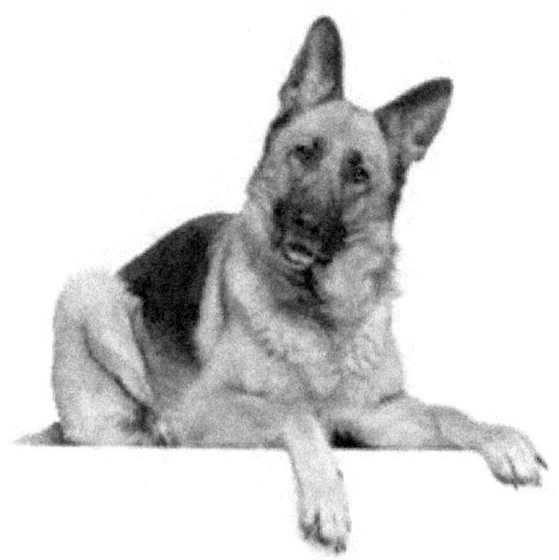

History:

German Shepherds are a generally new type of canine, having been reared late in the nineteenth century in Germany. They were rapidly conveyed to America, and utilized by both sides amid both World Wars. They could track foe aromas, and were additionally utilized as a part of mine location. Today, they are the most widely recognized police pooch. Their astounding responsiveness to orders and phenomenal faculties of smell make them flawless mates for their use in forces.

Tips:

German Shepherds are best if appropriately prepared. Their certainty is a characteristic attribute, and they will stand up beside or before their proprietors even with lazy proprietors. Ensure your Shepherd has a set bed; it is not prescribed to give your puppy a chance to rest in your bed, as it will comprehend this as his bed, and it will be exceptionally hard to have him move out. German Shepherds are exceptionally enthusiastic to learn, and will be excited to take charge and demonstrate its proprietor the amount it has learned. With legitimate tolerance and adoration, raising a German shepherd is entirely mellow contrasted with most breeds, and they have generally few wellbeing issues. There would not be a superior dog breed on the planet at securing your family, and flourishing around grown-ups and kids alike.

2.   Rottweiler:

The Rottweiler, if not appropriately prepared, is excessively forceful of a breed, making it impossible to have around little kids. Be that as it may, if appropriately prepared, this is surely one of the best choices for securing a family and their home. They are depicted to be one of the most brilliant pooch breeds on the planet, and can be prepared to be phenomenal gatekeeper canines. This is one breed we urge to have professionally prepared. The Rottweiler is awesome with families if raised appropriately, and even little kids are sheltered under the right conditions. Their insight can make them exceptionally submissive and regardless of their forceful growl, these puppies are extremely adoring and prepared to-please creatures.

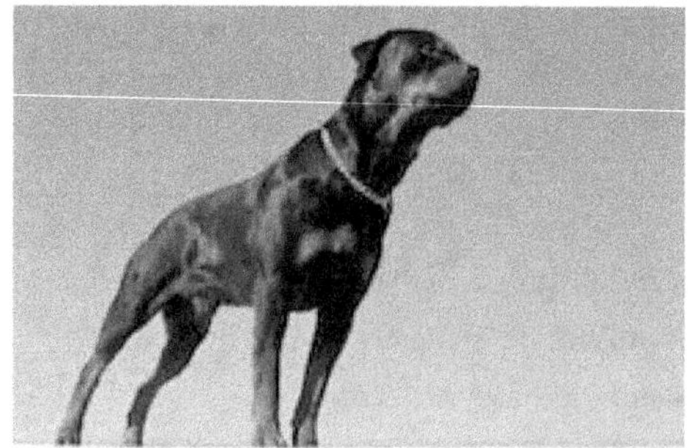

History:

This breed of Rottweiler was utilized by the Roman armed force as a part of times of war to secure the armed forces while they rested, and assault when in fight. In later years, this current breed's knowledge and forceful conduct made them incredible police pooches. They have been utilized for individual security as a part of both home settings, and assurance in travel.

Tips:

The requirement for concentrated and careful preparing can't be exaggerated. They are astute, and their regular impulses make them need to be pioneers. They have a fabulous wellbeing history, and are inclined to not very many maladies. Their greatest concern is tumor, yet that is inalienable in most puppy breeds. Their encouraging ought to be checked, and in the event that they are excessively worked out, their forcefulness tends to turn out. In home settings, these pooches flourish and are both faithful and steadfast and make extraordinary family dogs.

3.   Bullmastiff:

Bullmastiff has magnificent impulses and flourishes in family settings, as they learn rapidly who their "pack" is and will do all that they can to secure it. They are exceptionally mindful of everything going ahead around them, and their scary look settles on them an extraordinary decision at fighting off interlopers without putting your youngsters at danger. While some watchman canines will snarl and bark, if undermined, the Bullmastiff will indicate awesome assaulting qualities and can without much of a stretch take a full-developed man to the ground. All things considered, once it is acquainted with its home and who it's family is, this breed is tender and adoring, and will do extraordinary at being a piece of your family.

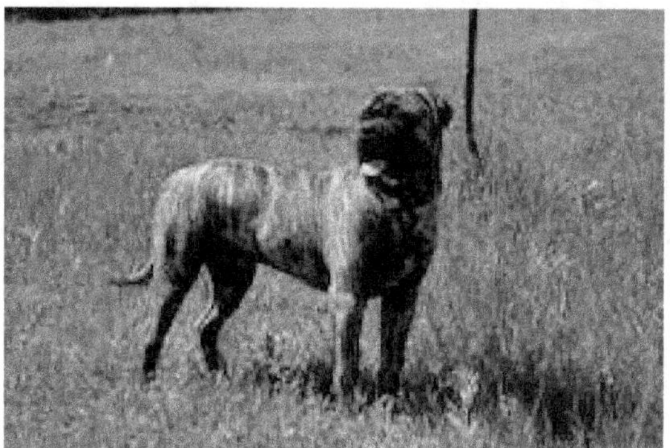

History:

As their name infers, the Bullmastiff is a blend of a bulldog and a mastiff. It was initially reared in England and was an awesome tracker, particularly during the evening. It worked unobtrusively, and made short work of most escapees and lawbreakers. They inevitably moved from wandering outside to being principally tamed, and flourished because of their devoted nature and attachment to their proprietors.

Tips:

Bullmastiffs, as most puppies on this rundown, should be prepared early and should be raised as a subordinate. Latent proprietors will lose control of their Bullmastiff, and it will overwhelm the home with little respect to summon and heading. If not raised appropriately, this breed does not do well with different breeds, as should be obvious different creatures as dangers and will snarl and bark. In spite of the fact that they are not inclined to numerous wellbeing issues,

Bullmastiffs regularly acquire hip and joint issues, and once in a while have issues with heart issues. They require regular activity, and also a solid.

4.   Doberman Pincher:

Doberman Pinchers are amazingly steadfast and exceptionally very much tuned to their proprietors summons if appropriately prepared. Pinchers are an incredible size, exceptionally coordinated and athletic. The breed is exceptionally ready and wary of individuals it is not acquainted with. Their snarl and bark are similarly scary, and interlopers will surely reconsider before entering your home. They ought to be brought up in the family with kids and not carried into a house with little kids after they are puppies.

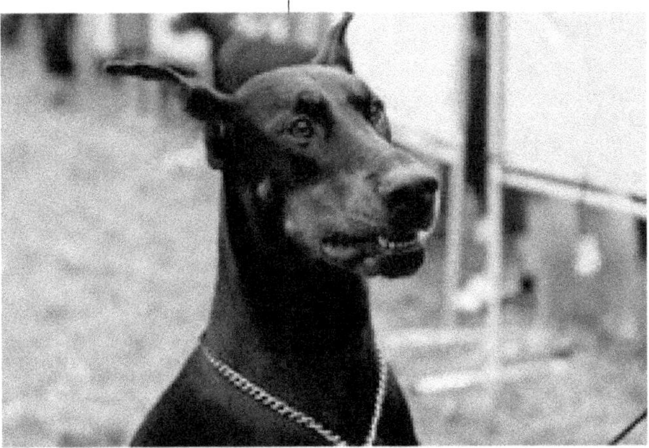

History

The Pincher was initially reared in Germany around the turn of the twentieth century. They were reproduced to be gatekeeper puppies, and have kept up those senses today. The Pincher was reared from an extensive variety of breeds, yet is accepted to most nearly look like greyhounds and terriers. This blend gives them their incredible physicality and faithful mentality. They were conveyed once more from Germany to the United States after World War 2 and have been utilized as a part of police and military circumstances up right up 'til the present time, however as of late; they have been utilized less and less as a part of these parts.

Tips:

Doberman Pinchers are shorthaired breeds that require minimal more than activity and sustenance to flourish in a home. They can be hard to prepare, and should be ruled at an early age to build up control and order of these canines for the duration of their lives. Their lifespan is moderately short; however they don't have numerous wellbeing issues on the off chance that they have routine vet checks. Their tails and ears likewise ought to be cut for wellbeing reasons.

Chapter 5 – Focus on the Security of Your Children and Disabled Family Members

Our family is at the focal point of our own universe. We would do practically anything for our family including shielding them from known peril and mischief. This can be troublesome on the grounds that we can't be with our kids at all times and we live in an open society where they can be presented to predators and vicious lawbreakers. The main spot where we have some control over our surroundings is in our home. We can make our home sensibly safe by strengthening it and equipping ourselves with self-preservation strategies important to ensure our family.

At whatever point a relative leaves the home, they leave the zone of insurance that we have made. One approach to keep our family sensible safe is to have a family security arrangement. At the point when building up a family security arrangement you should give cautious thought to the general population schedules of every relative and consider approaches to keep them safe. One approach to perform this is to hold a family meeting to talk about the security arrange and investigate consider the possibility that situations of genuine circumstances.

However, to secure your homes from thugs and thieves, certain approaches are used. Yet it is difficult to secure children and disabled people of house. Therefore, make sure of the following points to ensure the safety of your children and disabled family members:

- Guide them about the sudden exits of houses during the house meetings. Create a simple and easily understandable exit for them

- Play out a review of your front entryway, as well as all entryways around your home. Ensure the edges are solid, the pivots are secured, the wood is not empty, and, if your entryway has a mail opening, that somebody can't reach through it to open the entryway. The front entryway may be a decent point of convergence of your home, however don't give up security for a pretty view. On the off chance that your entryway doesn't have a peephole or a deadbolt, you ought to introduce those quickly to make the entryway considerably more secure.

- All homes ought to have some type of security framework, whether it's an essential camera establishment or a completely observed brilliant framework. Assess the requirements for your range and pick a framework you're alright with. A portion of the nuts and bolts to think about incorporate as an alert, movement sensors for the entryways and windows, and carbon monoxide and smoke finders.

- Your neighbors can be a useful first line of guard against a home attack. They know the zone and can watch out for your home when you're away — yet they can't do that in the event that they don't have any acquaintance with you. Endeavor to meet your new neighbors and frame great connections so you will have individuals to depend on. In the event that something fishy is going on in your general vicinity, a great neighbor will call and let you know.

\-   Discover data on reaching the nearby police, check for an area watch program, and see what different assets your region has accessible to help in home security. Some neighborhood police strengths will send an officer over to provide you with tips for securing your house. Moreover, keep these numbers on your recent dials. This will help the disabled members and children to call at these numbers with ease.

Conclusion

To put in a nutshell, this book incorporates a thorough examination about how to secure your home from threats and dangers. With a specific approach to answer this question, this book incorporates different aspects about how to annihilate this risk and secure your home. Hence, this book gives endless supply of tips and methods that guarantee security.

Firstly, arranging the fundamental security is the most vital thing to give prosperous and safe life. Thus, this book incorporates certain strategies about essential security arrangements. Secondly, physical protection is among the most vital methods that can help you secure yourself from a wide range of dangers. Therefore, a guide is provided in this book to achieve this approach. Moreover, the significance of learning the technique of physical defense is explained. Thirdly, the vital arsenals to secure your home are likewise elaborated in the text. Fourthly, tips about keeping guard dogs are included to help the reader in the training process. In the end, another vital viewpoint i.e. systems to secure the youngsters and disabled individuals is likewise included the coming content.

In this way, this combination of systems for security of your home and family is a book worth-reading. It not just serves as a manual for home security, but also, it incorporates in itself the insights about the significance of these strategies. Additionally, the safety oriented measures that must be embraced by the people are likewise another astonishing part of this book. In this manner, this book empowers a man to take in the procedures required for a safe home.

Ham Radio

Introduction

Since the evolution of mankind, mankind has been busy in inventing new technology for their own ease and comfort. In every domain of life humans are seeking to develop novel technology which is obviously better than its previous invention.

With expansion of cities and communities around the world humans had felt a need to develop communication between cities for trade or business. In early days man is send as messenger so he would have to travel hundreds of miles just to deliver a message which is time consuming and hectic thing to do so researchers from around the world started thinking about solving this issue and hence the milestone called radio was achieved.

The journey starts with an Italian scientist Guglielmo Marconi who gave the idea of signal transmission by practically demonstrating a telegraph sent from long distance over a radio signals in late 19th century. Later on in early 90's concept of radio was introduced and soon it became main source of news broadcasting and communication between long distances.

From idea of radio a thought emerged about setting up a radio anywhere you want. In late 90's radio was used for entertainment, news and other purposes so with variety of things it can deal in, it gives a pleasure to number of people to operate, setup and develop their own radios in their place. This concept gave birth to a concept called "Ham Radio "The first ever occasion in which ham radio was practically used is Christmas Eve of 1906 and a Christmas story was broadcast named as "silent night" in Bible.

Chapter 1 – Overview of Ham Radio and High Frequency Communications

Ham radio:

Amateur radio are also called as ham radio and beginners in radio operation are referred as hams. It can be adopted as a hobby as it was a trendy hobby in late 90's in USA. Even today we can see a lot of people using ham radio on commercial and individual level.

Hams and their interest:

Ham radio attract practitioners with a good vary of interests. Several amateurs begin with a fascination of radio communication which then develops into a hobby. A number of the focal areas hams adopt radio contesting, radio broadcast study, public service communication (PSC), technical experimentation and laptop networking.

Ham radio operators use numerous modes of transmission to speak. The two most typical modes for voice transmissions are:

- Area unit modulation (FM)

- Single sideband (SSB)

FM offers prime quality audio signals, whereas SSB is healthier at long distance communication once information measure is restricted. The amateur radio service (amateur service and amateur-satellite service) or service in setting up a ham is established by the International Telecommunication Union (ITU) through the International Telecommunication rules. National governments regulate technical associate in nursing the operational characteristics of transmissions and issue individual stations licenses with a unique decision sign. These beginner operators are tested for his or her understanding of key ideas in natural philosophy and also the host government's radio rules.

Radio amateurs use a spread of voice, text, image, and information communications modes and have access to frequency allocations throughout the RF spectrum to alter communication across a town, region, country, continent, the world, or maybe into area.

Every year, hams round the world participate in an occasion designed to bolster the power to setup and operate a good station victimization emergency power and temporary antennas, throughout a weekend long event referred to as Field Day.

High Frequency:

It is basically range of electromagnetic waves or radio waves between ranges of 3 to 30 MHz, it is used to provide noise free channels that enables smooth communication between transfer and receiver.

High frequency Communications:

High Frequency spectrum is used in molding communication system that benefits physical properties of the HF Radio Channel.

Using high frequency for communication:

- It's greatest worth is its ability to produce reliable short AND long-range on the far side Line Of Sight (BLOS) communications.

- It is reliable and needs little infrastructure to build up.

- It supports point-to point and point to multipoint conversations with less likelihood of noise in channels.

Ham radios and communication:

Amateur radio is independent of terrestrial facilities that may fail. It is distributed throughout community and there are no "choke points" or noise in channels like radio telephone sites.

 Ham radios can be utilize for functions of non-commercial exchange of messages, wireless experimentation, self-training, non-public recreation, radio sport, contesting, and emergency communication.

For example you are on a trip or vacation with your school and to add some fun and excitement you can setup your own ham radio on spot and you can broadcast messages or song dedication etc. on your radio which will enlighten up the environment indeed.

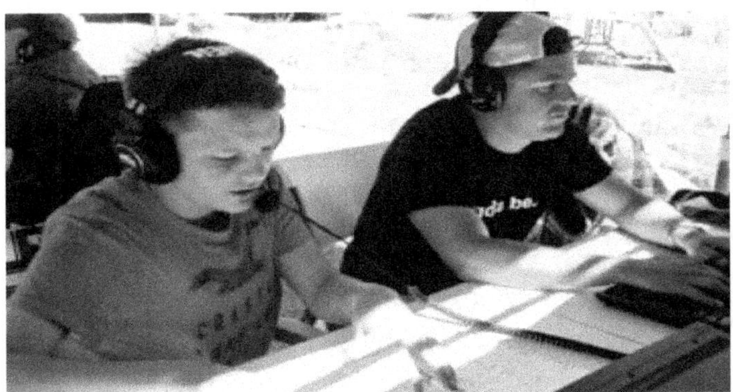

More over ham radios can also be used as a key in disaster management. In case of any disaster or emergency you can set up a ham radio to boost up communication between victims and helpers.

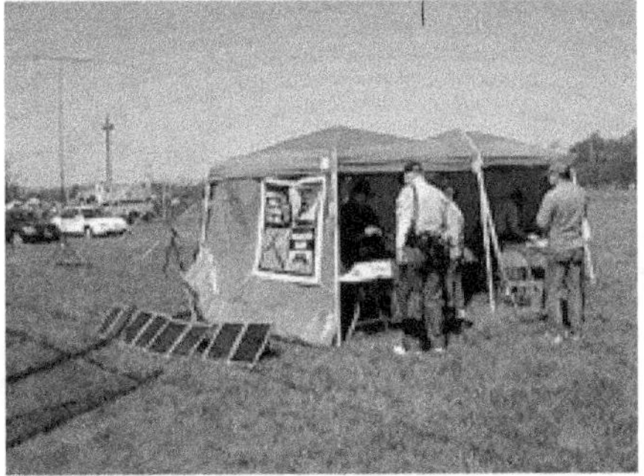

An important example of "ham radio" is its use by New York City agencies to keep in touch with each other after their command center was destroyed during the 9/11 incident. Ham radio also came as a tool for disaster management during natural disasters like Hurricane Katrina, where all other communications failed, and also in the devastating flooding in Colorado in 2013.

There are few Intimidations that could be faced by hams or ham radios:

Attempted spectrum grabs, wherever enticing bands allotted to amateurs become vulnerable by industrial and alternative interests that need the precious spectrum, sporadically rear their head. Bands that are in demand, the 70cm band, was recently granted a keep of execution. Broadband over Power line (BPL), associate unrelated future technology that uses utility lines to supply web access, has the potential to cause interference and trim back from Amateur Radio Ham signals, in line with Major Ham cluster ARRL. There square measure people who dispute this.

Chapter 2 – Key Concepts of Ham Radio

Hams:

The operators of ham can also be called as hams. There is no specific qualification required for being ham but it requires some skill and knowledge of radio along with keen interest in this domain. Ham Radio operators are missionaries, celebrities, students, doctors, politicians, truck drivers or regular folks hence they can be people from all fields of life. There are number of legal talented young ham Radio operators currently than it was in previous times.

Ham radio significance:

Hams or Ham Radio is the kind aptitude to speak across the road, country or even worldwide, or perhaps with satellites, space stations in space or individual level. Even if there is no electricity, and also the cell phones and landlines are not working, with few equipment like a wire, a radio, and a battery, ham radio is there to use. Ham Radio enables North American nation relish their life-long distant friends, and an active technical activity or education. It boosts up the motivation, resources and encourages to experiment and play with new equipment's. It also encourages ham to adopt new styles that are governed by novel technology and newest way of communicating things.

You can't say that the sky is that the limit once there area unit footprints on the moon! You'll be able to go anyplace you wish, without boundary lines, and amateur radio will assist you get there!

Some major concepts that has to be kept in mind while setting up or talking about ham radio are:

- Skills that should be possessed by operators. They should have keen interest in ham radio along with particular set of skills.

- You should have license to operate radio in any place you want. Most hams have United States license and its validity last for 10 years.

- The next important thing is antenna, its setting location and many other factors concerning its performance.

- Purpose of ham is also an important aspects. You can either use it for personal or commercial purposes and you can also use it in emergency cases or in medical relief camps etc.

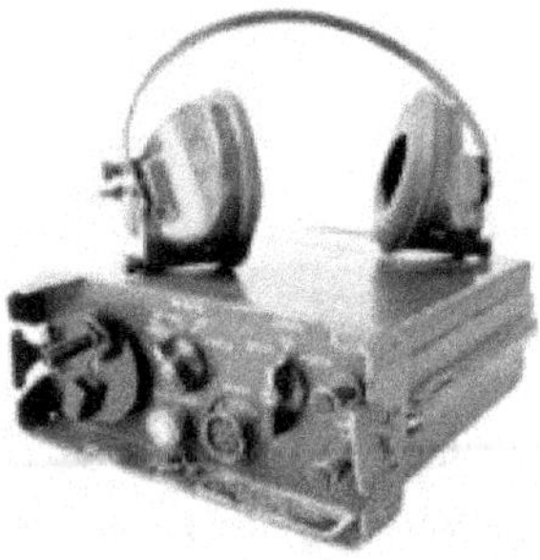

Hams square measure at the leading edge of the many technologies. They supply thousands of hours of volunteer community and emergency services once traditional communications go down or square measure overladen. All of them fancy being creators, not simply shoppers, of wireless technology.

Types of Ham Radios

There are three types of ham radios:

- **Handheld:**

Small and light-weight, hand-held transceivers enable ham operators to speak on the go; as a result of their low power output, hand-held ham radios generally have variety of solely five miles at the most; their range may be inflated by a close-by ham radio repeater.

- **Mobility:**

Designed to be used from associate operator's vehicle or a ham shack; their 200-mile vary is usually as a result of the raised power out there through either a home wall association or by an association through a vehicle's battery via a 12-volt outlet or power adapter.

- **Base station**

Designed to be used from associate operator's vehicle or a ham shack; their 200-mile vary is sometimes as a results of the raised power out there through either a home wall association or by an association through a vehicle's battery via a 12volt outlet or power adapter.

Some fun facts about ham radio:

- There are approximately a total of 50,000 radio hams in North American nation.

- There aren't any age or status constraints applying to people who consent for Canadian amateur radio license.

- There square measure Amateur Radio clubs attending nearly each group.

- Morse code is not any longer needed so as to get Basic Amateur Radio Certification.

Multi domain purpose:

- **Education:**

Self-education. It polishes your skills for broadcasting. It can also be adopted as field of education. Helping another pursuing knowledge and skills, are traditions in Amateur Radio. Once you have legal rights and authorization you never stop learning.

- **Intercommunication:**

Hams exercise communicating in groups or "networks" and individually on a regular basis to acquire practical expertise in interacting "traffic" under all circumstances.

- **Excellent Platform for all amateurs:**

It provides an efficient interactive system for hams around the world to contact each other and gather whole hams community on one common platform in friendly environment. This will boost up their knowledge and skills.

- **Public Service**:

It can be used for serving public in variety of ways. Ham radios offer communication during simulated or real emergencies, and for noncommercial occasions.

- **Experimentation:**

Within the framework of the Radio communication Act, amateurs with frequency allocations and license can experiment with new modes and techniques of radio communication. This will develop new methods and techniques for hams.

Chapter 3 – Tips to get Ham Radio License

Since radio instrumentation has the potential to interfere with alternative radio transmissions, operators should learn some info concerning radio, however it works, and therefore the rules governing amateur radio. There accustomed be six license categories within the North American nation, however that has a lot of recently been reduced to three: Technician, General, and Extra. Every future category needs a lot of data and grants additional privileges with regards to permissible transmission bands.

So the first thing you need to do before going to broad cast your channel or something on ham radio , you need to get your license and you should be aware of the terms and conditions for legally operating a ham radio. Here I have discussed few tips that would guide you how to get your license.United States license is worldwide known so I will be discussing about its classes and pre requirements in getting your license.

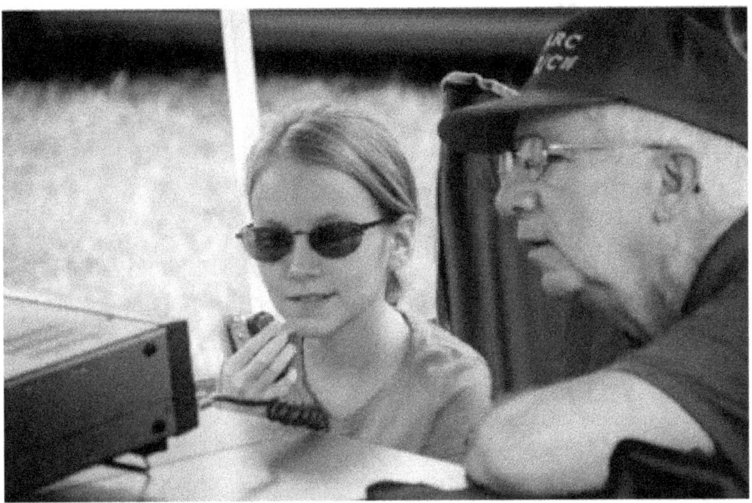

Ham radio license in United States

In US, amateur radio licensing is authorized by Federal Communications commission (FCC) underneath strict federal guidelines. Licenses to operate newbie stations for non-public usage is granted to individuals of any age when they show an interest in understanding of each pertinent of FCC policies and expertise of radio station operation and safety concerns.

Candidates as young as five years antique have exceeded examinations and have been granted licenses. December 2012 marked one hundred years of beginner radio operator and station licensing with the aid of the United States authorities.

Operator licenses are divided into distinctive training, each one of which corresponds to a growing degree of expertise and corresponding privileges. With new era of technology, the info of the instructions have modified drastically, leading to the modern gadget of open instructions. License validity last for 10 years and then operator have to renew his license.

License classes in US

The FCC classifications of licensing have evolved notably because of the software's inception. Whilst the FCC made the maximum changes recently. It has allowed positive existing operator training to stay beneath a grandfather clause. Those licenses would not be issued to new candidates, however present licenses may be changed or renewed indefinitely after period of 10 years. More over if any individual other than us citizen who wants to have US amateur radio license can appear in an exam conducted by volunteer examiners. It is conducted on monthly basis.

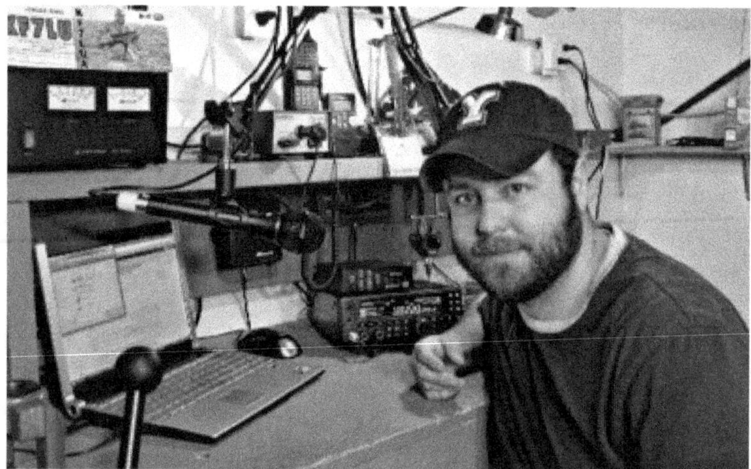

The two classes of ham radio are discussed below:

- **Novice classes**

The novice classes' magnificence operator license turned into for operators who had exceeded a five phrase in line with minute (wpm) Morse code examination and a basic idea exam. After the 1987 restructuring, privileges covered 4 bands inside the HF ranges 3–30 MHz, one band inside the Very High Frequency (VHF) varies from 30–three hundred MHz, and one band within the ultra-high frequency (UHF) ranges from 300–3,000MHz. This class became deprecated with the aid of the restructuring in 2000. novice operators received Morse code most effective privileges inside the entire Morse code and information simplest segments of the general magnificence quantities of eighty, forty, 15 and information and Morse code inside the general section of 10 meters in 2007 simply prior to the Morse code requirement.

- **Advance class**

The advanced magnificence operator license, whose privileges have intently resemblance with general class license, however covered 275 kHz of additional spectrum in the HF bands, changed into deprecated by the restructuring in 2000.

Ham radio types:

There are three types of ham radio. These are as follow:

- **Technician:**

The entry-level licensing alternative, giving access to any or all of the ham radio frequencies on top of thirty megahertz; these frequencies area unit found in North America specifically with restricted shortwave access to locations abroad.

- **General**

The next grade from amateur radio licenses is that the General license and needs operators to pass the technician level license needs first; this license provides access to any or all amateur radio bands and sets the user   up for worldwide communication.

- **Amateur further**

The highest of all 3 licenses; needs users to pass each the Technician License take a look at and therefore the General License take a look at, giving the operator access to any or all operative privileges each abroad and within the U.S.

Chapter 4 – Tips to set an Antenna and set a Station

A radio antenna is the critical hyperlink in any receiving or transmitting station whether or not it is used for ham radio, quick wave listening, or for industrial or professional use. The general performance of the radio station depends upon the overall performance of the radio antenna. An efficient radio antenna will enable the overall performance of the whole radio communications station to be maximum, whereas a poor antenna will degrade the competencies of the transmitter and receiver no matter how correct they are.

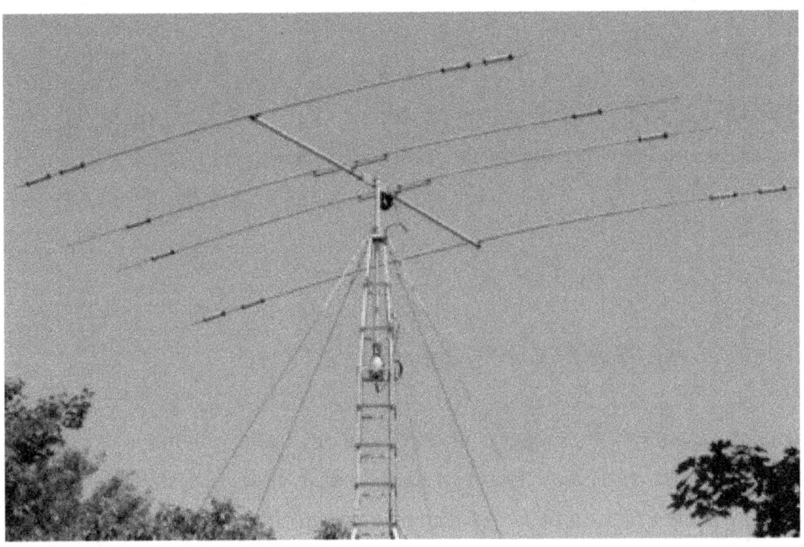

Radio stations used for professional or business packages have a big share in reliable performance. They may site antennas in which they may give a suitable level of performance but for ham radio enthusiasts or people who have adopted it as a hobby and brief wave listeners it's far essential to put it in the high-quality antenna around the residence.

Only a few ham radio operators are able to utilize an area or other huge location, and frequently the radio antenna might be something of a compromise. However, via following some hints, it's far feasible to make the excellent of any radio antenna set up and make sure that its performance is as true as possible further to this it's far worth citing that it also includes important to adopt some experimentation to find out what type of radio antenna works satisfactory for a given place and fashion of radio operation.

A few pointers and guidelines are given below for your ease, but these can simplest be general pointers, and they're now not exhaustive. However they shape a terrific beginning place when deliberating installing a ham radio antenna machine.

General settings of an antenna for ham radio:

One of the most vital components of putting in any radio antenna is its vicinity. The region of the antenna will govern many aspects of its operation, and therefore the vicinity of the antenna ought to be determined alongside the kind of antenna to be used.

Some of factors associated with the antenna must be considered:

- Pick an area in which the radio antenna can "see" all around: in order for to operate at its best it have to be capable of "see" all round it. So that you can achieve this it need to be kept far from nearby objects that could act as a screen. In this manner the maximum amount of sign can be attain or go away the antenna without being absorbed in close by gadgets.

- Secondly keep in mind that nearby gadgets can "detune" an antenna: whilst thinking about the location of a radio antenna it is really worth remembering that close by gadgets can detune an antenna despite the fact that they do no longer have an effect on the all spherical visibility.

- Surrounded gadgets can purpose an antenna to operate away from its resonant factor and become much less green. It can be very critical for antennas which might be cut to a particular length and do no longer have a means of being tuned in situ. Many items can motive this to show up - steel gadgets in addition to electric wiring are mainly horrific however even trees can degrade the performance of antennas in this way. Typically the consequences are important inside distances of a wavelength or the nearer the object and the more the conductivity the greater the effect.

- Another fact keep in mind appropriate points for anchoring antennas: Horizontal antennas want anchor factors at either stop. This is worth thinking about whether there are any appropriate anchor factors already in lifestyles. Chimneys or different points on the residence can provide one suitable point.

- Trees will also be positioned with no trouble, even though pulley schemes are required to permit any motion in the tree because of wind to be taken up without snapping the antenna twine. Additionally it may be feasible to erect a pole or antenna mast and attention can be given to this possibility and its vicinity. Anything alternative is decided upon, this must be considered at the outset.

- Inner or out: frequently the use of an internal radio antenna may also need to be taken into consideration. Outside antennas function higher because they may be in addition faraway from gadgets on the way to introduce loss or detune the antenna. It is very tough to estimate the quantity of loss which having an antenna in the house has. The roof or brickwork will motive the sign to be reduced, in particular while it's far moist. The amount of loss can even depend on the frequency. For VHF and UHF indicators this can be a whole lot greater.

- Some other factors that should be observed while setting an antenna are antenna height, matching of antenna with feeder, safety aspects of antenna, consideration of feeders that enables maximum power transmitted by an antenna.

Chapter 5 – Learn how to set up a Ham Radio?

Owning and in operation a ham radio, or amateur radio, offers people a fun and rewarding hobby or perhaps how to speak throughout a crisis. Operators should make sure that their rig is setup properly, and that they should additionally become licensed for in operation a ham radio before use. Being knowledgeable within the use of a ham radio parades a world of prospects to operators, permitting them to speak with other people and even permits them to speak regionally throughout emergency situations.

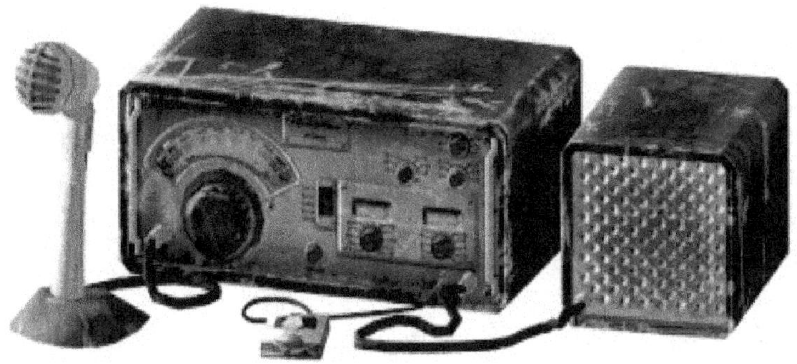

To get the foremost use out of owning and in operation a ham radio, house, owners have to be compelled to perceive all of the choices and options that the communication system has got to provide. They ought to even be accustomed to the various sorts of ham radios, common brands, what the necessities square measure to work a ham radio, and places to seek out and get ham radios, like at native physical science stores or on-line marketplaces like eBay. So, to get pleasure from the system within the trendy age, it is important to be told concerning frequency sorts, sorts of licenses, parts of a ham radio, and therefore the advantages of in operation a ham radio.

There is an important aspect to preserve in thoughts. Ham radio is an exquisite food for many people who have adopted it as a hobby. There are nearby emergency infrastructures (which we're organizing up radios for in this sequence) besides this there are other complete-direction meals concerning extreme Frequency communications where low energy activists (like me) want to check that how many states round the sector will "work" in Morse code. Morse code isn't obligatory for a ham authorization any longer, but that's another thing.

Digital modes are also there. Some operators enjoy doing sluggish-scan TV – directing photographs to Europe or anyplace, as any other complete meal with the aid of itself. The "guides" in that one take account of virtual images, transmitter techniques, photograph-shopping, in addition to "ordinary" High Frequency radio usage.

This entry-stage path is one step, but at hand are loads. There's a ham station involved the transnational area Station, and "running" Japan the usage of nothing extra than a Very High Frequency (VHF) radio and a hand-held directional small beam antenna, is a full "subsequent meal" for some.

Elmer:

In amateur radio, the term "Elmer" refers to a mentor, or to the act of mentoring others. This is often integral to the ham radio spirit of serving to others. Several more-experienced hams can volunteer their time to answer queries, give tutoring or teach categories to anyone desire to enter amateur radio ranks, or World Health Organization merely needs to be told additional regarding it.

The amateur radio community could be a various network of clubs and people like an expert in an exceedingly type of areas. For some, sharing or business enterprise sensible data is their approach of giving back to the ham radio community.

There square measure several engineering and scientific professionals concerned in ham radio still as several celebrities. Journalist director Cronkite, baseball pitcher Bokkos Swobada, TV/radio temperament Jean Shepherd, legislator Barry Goldwater, and musician Joe Walsh square measure among the thousands of notable personalities World Health Organization square measure or were hams. Honor winner for Physics Joseph Taylor is a fanatical ham, and has developed many modulation formats that square measure appropriate for very weak signal communications.

Components of Ham Radio:

- **Shake:**

It depicts the location from where ham radio would be operated

- **Antenna:**

It is used to catch signals

- **Cables:**

These are used to connect transceiver with antenna and to make other wired connections

- **Guide wires:**

These wires helps in stabilizing of antenna.

- **Power supply:**

Provides power to equipment's of ham radio

- **Fuses:**

It protects electric equipment from power damage.

- **Battery:**

It is used to give current supply to antenna and other equipment.

- **Transceiver:**

It is used to receive signals

- **Antenna tuner:**

It helps in improving antenna capacity to catch signals efficiently.

- **Antenna rotator:**

Rotates antenna in different direction so that signals are catch accurately.

Setting up a ham:

First, if you're a Maker, then you have already got lots in you not unusual with the ham radio network. Hams are tinkerers, developers, fixers, and inventors by means of nature. As an Entrepreneur in this field, the field (or building your own field) is not most effective allowed, it's advocated! Of the numerous radio services obtainable from business broadcasting to Commercial purposes to public protection.

Amateur radio is the handiest one in which gadget may be home made and tuned to any frequency or channel that hams have access to. Flexibility, experimentation, and hacking are a way of existence with hams. Ham radio has many aspects it's absolutely 1000 interests in a single. You can dive deeply into electronics, antennas, digital communications, public service, competitive working, solar and geophysics technology, global-extensive "DX-ing," or just use ham radio as a private communications tool.

A few hams attention on just one or a few topics while others try and enjoy it all! As a Maker, you're in all likelihood maximum interested in the electronics, however once you begin digging in, you never understand in which it would lead or where you could apply your talents.

Whilst they're at the air, hams use dozens of different sorts of alerts; some are everyday voice indicators wherein we certainly talk to each other and yes some hams use Morse code at the same time as others are designing their very own virtual protocols to send statistics and messages around the world. Hams have their very own e mail and data networks. There are even ham radio satellites that relay signals, such as a ham station at the worldwide space Station that the astronauts use — they're hams, too. Hams perform from their homes, their cars, and even from mountaintops and islands!

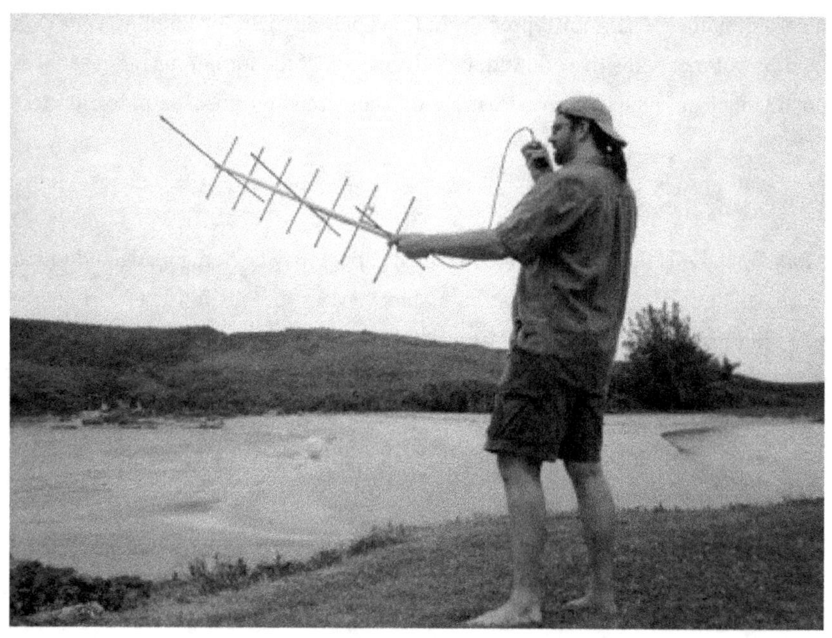

All that equipment sounds highly-priced, but it doesn't must be. much like beginning your own workshop, you may preserve it simple, purchase used gear, scrounge for elements and portions, and work with different extra experienced hams (we call the mentors Elmer) to get started. The only access-degree radios fee much less than a hundred dollar and you can build your personal antenna.

Loose software program is extensively available on the way to use some of the distinctive sorts of signals, even Morse code which hams talk over with as "CW" for continuous wave. So, a primary radio, a couple of cables, and also you're in commercial enterprise to start as a novice ham. Just get concerned, search for funny-looking antennas, and ask around. You'll be amazed how pleasant, fun loving and helpful a few hams are!

Conclusion:

Concluding the description I can say that Ham radios afford their operators the chance to get involved in with folks worldwide that they might unremarkably check with and share common interests and new concepts with others.

In associate degree emergency state of affairs, ham radios additionally permit their operators to speak with authorities to function a possible resource in those styles of things at intervals in their community. Ham radios area unit still helpful within the fashionable age thanks to their ability to still work even once different varieties of communication don't seem to be. Operators additionally fancy opportunities to move and even hold contests for contacting the foremost users in an exceedingly given period of time.

Adopting it as a hobby is another interesting way to get in touch with this fully loaded piece of invention. Even if a person is interested in electronics or media stuff he can begin his practical training by setting up a ham radio. It is indeed skill building practice.

For those that decide that in operation a ham radio continues to be helpful, they'll get the instrumentation at numerous locations, however ought to be bear in mind to get a license before causation any messages. Before shopping for a ham radio, bear in mind to analyze accessible choices and study the various styles of ham radios, the necessities to awfully operate one, and the way to shop for ham radios safely and firmly on eBay.

It's conjointly serving to build basic skills that aren't any longer tutored at school rising not solely our ability to speak in disasters, however adding back a number of the 'lost tools' that Americans accustomed be notable for the power to try and do things ourselves. You will find this text utterly useful and compre-hendible. I am 100% sure that with your interest, knowledge and guideline from this text you can surely setup your own ham radio.

Harvest Wild Meat: 15 Simple Traps and Snares

Introduction

You can find yourself in a situation of wilderness either by choice or by the circumstances of disaster or an emergency. Whatever the situation is, you need to acquire warmth, seeking rescue, finding plenty of drinkable water, providing shelter and edible food. The food is not that simple to get in the wild as not all of the sources are edible.

Many varieties of flora and fauna are found in the wild. All of them are good source of fat and protein such as insects, worms, mammals, reptiles, amphibians, crustaceans, mollusks, fish and birds. But not all species of these food sources are edible.

Also trapping and killing them is not easy in the wild. You need to get a little technical with the trapping and hunting techniques here but first you should know what you should hunt. Therefore, let's start by looking at the edible options available in the wild for your dinner menu.

Chapter 01: List of Safe and Unsafe Animals to Eat

It is always good to consider hunting small animals than to bait on the big game in the wilderness. Small animals are found abundantly in the wild. They are also easier to prepare and cook. But you may not all kinds of the animals that you can actually eat in the wild. Some of them are poisonous as well and not suitable as food. Here, we are discussing some of the animals that you can eat in the wild;

Insects:

The most abundant life forms found on the planet earth is that of the insects. They are big source of protein. This makes them an important food.

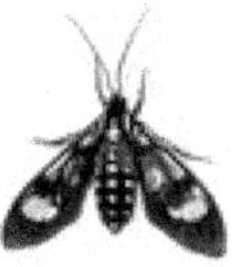

http://images.freeimages.com/images/thumbs/f96/black-and-red-insect-1409171.jpg

But there are a few insects that you must avoid to eat. They include all those types of insects that are adult, brightly colored, hairy or the ones that sting or bite. Also avoid caterpillars, spiders and all the kinds of insects that have a pungent odor. All kinds of common disease carriers such as mosquitoes, flies and ticks must also be avoided.

Worms:

Another good source of protein available in the wild is the worms. You can find them above the ground after rain or dig them down in the damp soil.

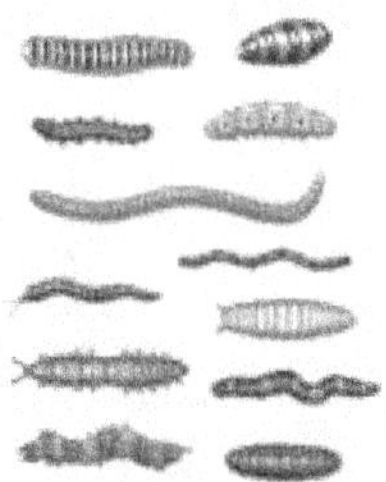

http://i.istockimg.com/file_thumbview_approve/34652434/3/stock-illustration-34652434-caterpillars-and-worms.jpg

Drop them in clean water as you capture the worms. Let them be in the portable water for a few minutes. The worms have a natural habit of purging. Therefore, they will clean themselves up in the water. You can eat them raw right afterwards.

Crustaceans:

Crayfish is abundantly found in the fresh water. It is akin to marine crabs and lobsters. To distinguish them from each other, check their five pairs of legs and hard exoskeleton. Also that the pair of their front legs have oversized pincers is another point of difference.

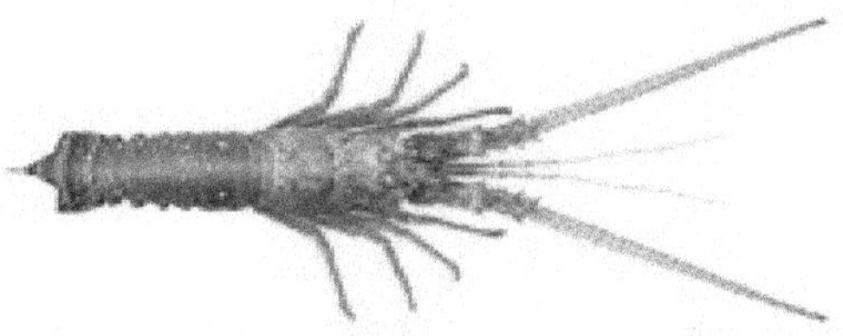

http://images.freeimages.com/images/thumbs/493/lobster-1322337.jpg

Fresh water shrimps are also a good source of food in the wild. Their size ranges from 0.25 to 2.5 centimeters. They usually form large colonies in mud bottoms of the lakes and ponds and in mats of floating algae.

You can also find shrimps, crabs and lobsters to 10 meter deep in the water. You may scoop the shrimps out of the water when they come to the surface at the night with the help of a net. However, you would have to use baits to catch crabs and lobsters. They are best caught at night.

Mollusks:

Saltwater and freshwater shellfish such as sea urchins, chitons, periwinkles, barnacles, bivalves, mussels, clams and snails and octopuses are all edible.

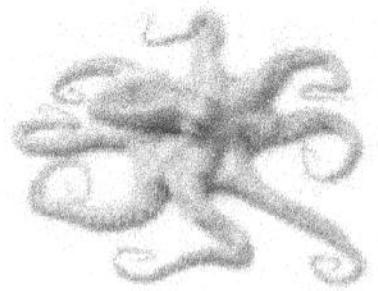

http://i.istockimg.com/file_thumbview_approve/16089264/3/stock-photo-16089264-whole-single-fresh-raw-octopus.jpg

In fresh water, they are found shallow water with muddy or sandy bottoms whereas in seas, they are commonly found in the wet sand and the tidal pools.

Fish:

Fish is an excellent source of fat and protein. They are usually abundantly found thus make a good food source. Catching fish is easier and there are a number of ways through which you can catch them.

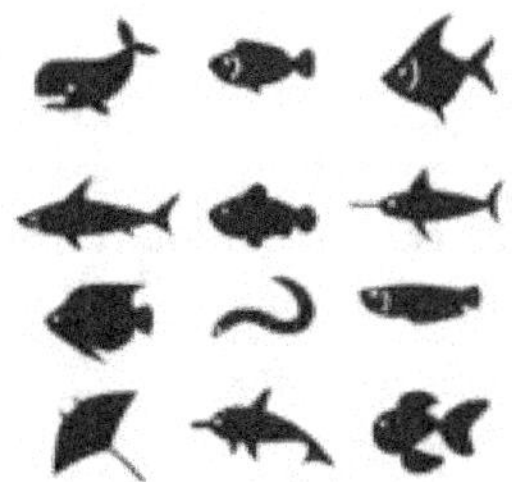

http://i.istockimg.com/file_thumbview_approve/75695091/3/stock-illustration-75695091-silhouette-fish-icon-set.jpg

No freshwater fish is poisonous. The catfish, however, have sharp protrusions on its dorsal barbells and fins. They can give you painful puncture wounds that can also easily get infected.

Amphibians:

Salamanders and frogs are easily found around the pools of fresh water. It is not easy to capture frogs however as they plunge deep into the water on the first sight of danger nearby. Salamanders are easily caught at night time.

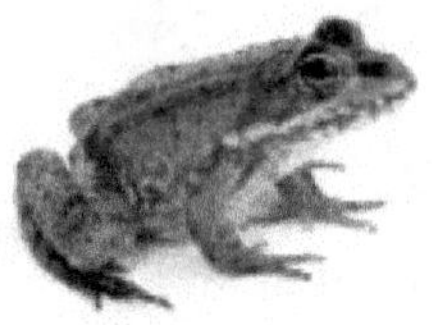

http://i.istockimg.com/file_thumbview_approve/2142843/3/stock-photo-2142843-green-frog.jpg

Some species of frogs are poisonous as well. It is good to avoid all kind of frogs with bright color of skins and a distinct X mark on their backs.

Reptiles:

Another good source of protein out there in the wild comes from reptiles. They are also easier to catch. You can even eat them raw however their raw meat may transfer parasites as they are cold blooded.

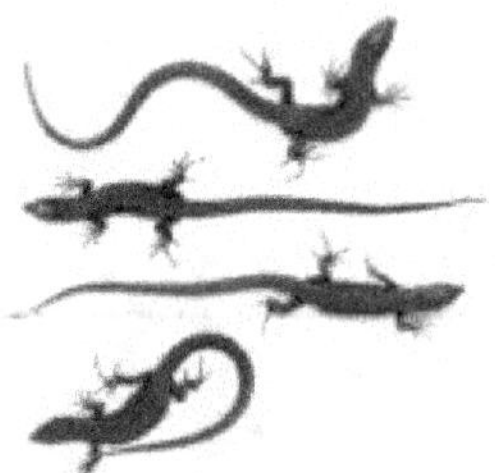

http://i.istockimg.com/file_thumbview_approve/14404686/3/stock-photo-14404686-lizard.jpg

Alligators, crocodiles, tortoises, turtles, lizards, and snakes are all reptiles. But you should never eat a box and hawksbill turtles. Also avoid poisonous large sea turtles, crocodiles, alligators and snakes.

Birds:

Good news is that birds are edible; all species of them! However, the flavors vary considerably. It is also easy to catch them and they are abundantly found too.

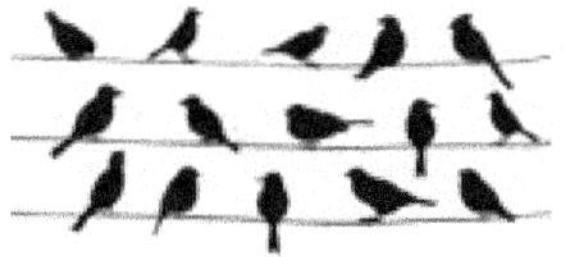

http://i.istockimg.com/file_thumbview_approve/77244301/3/stock-illustration-77244301-cute-black-birds-on-a-wire.jpg

Nesting birds also provide you with another food source and that is their eggs. You can eat the too.

Mammals:

Mammals are considered to be the tastiest source of food. There are certain drawbacks in catching them however. Like the number of wounds depend upon the size of the mammal. Also they can sense the snares and traps sometimes.

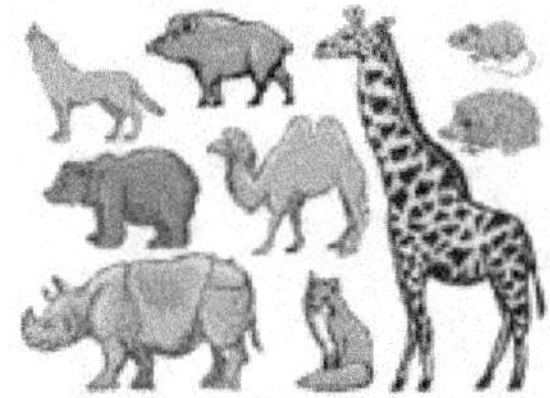

http://i.istockimg.com/file_thumbview_approve/46518806/3/stock-illustration-46518806-mammals.jpg

Chapter 02: Setting Snares for Small Games and Big Animals

Snares are the effective traps to catch small games and big animals. They are considered to be one among the very first traps used by human to harvest furbearers and small games. Modernized versions are used today. They are preferred over other types of traps because they are easy to make, light weight and can be carried to long distances in large numbers.

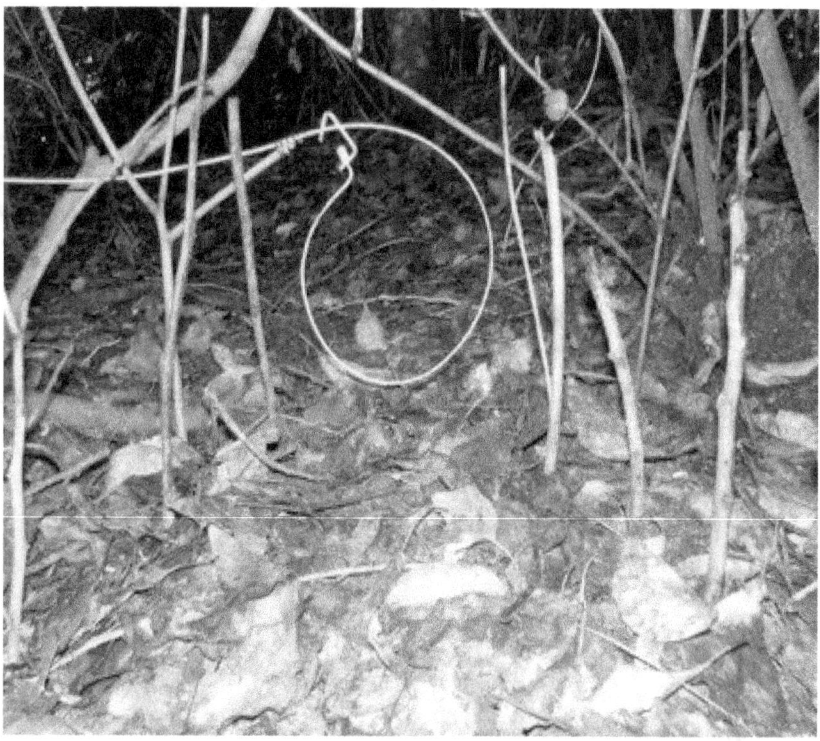

http://cdn.instructables.com/FAZ/OAVC/I0YGCTWS/FAZOAV-
CI0YGCTWS.MEDIUM.jpg

You can buy a readymade snare from the market but you can also make it yourself. It is very easy and for your interest, the detailed process is given as under;

Step # 01: Understanding How Snares Work:

Tightly wound steel cables are used to make snares these days. Thickness may vary but 3/32" is a good measurement to settle down. Keep the cable 5 to 7 feet in length.

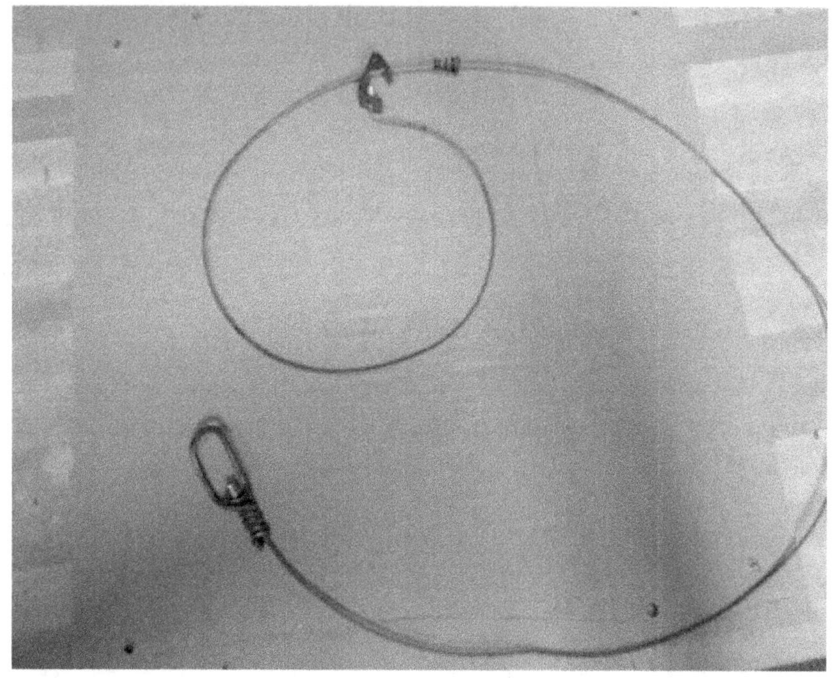

http://cdn.instructables.com/FFH/PE8G/I0YGCTVH/FFH-PE8GI0YGCTVH.MEDIUM.jpg

On their main loops, snares have one way locking system. It slides down on a small touch and gets tightened around the neck of the animal. A swivel is added at the end of the cable so the captured animal can move around freely without twisting and thus breaking the cable.

Step # 02: Anchoring Your Snare:

Best area to set your snare trap is where the target animal is found to be traveling frequently. Anchor your snare on the optimal location. Simply take a stiff wire and loop it through the swivel of the snare and tie it around any tree or any other solid object. You can use a coat hanger to tie the swivel with the tree as well.

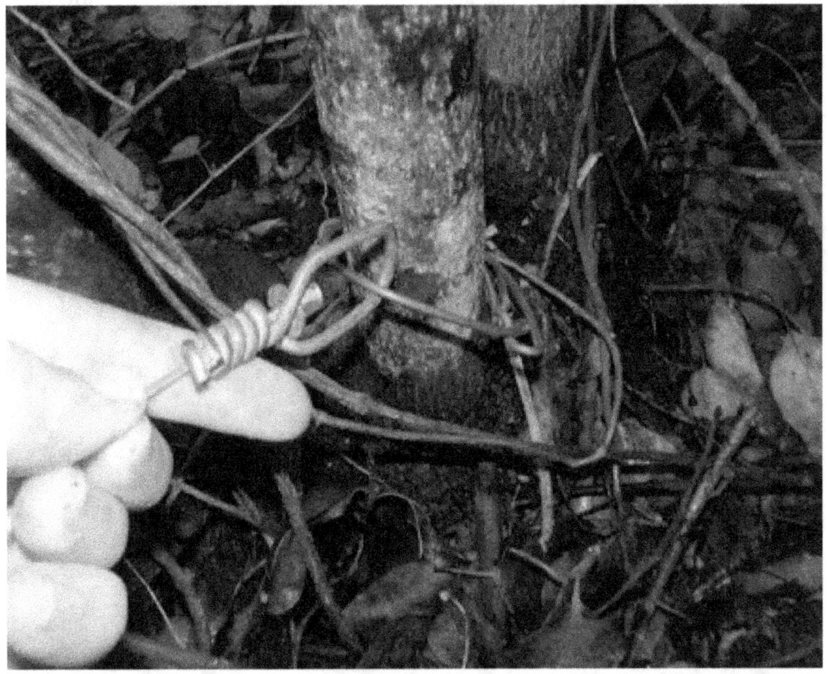

http://cdn.instructables.com/FVB/B6SK/I0YGCTVZ/FVB-B6SKI0YGCTVZ.MEDIUM.jpg

Once you have tied your snare, support it with the help of a stick and stand it in a position so that the targeted animal can move through the loop. The slight movement inside the loop will slide down the one way locking system and the animal will be trapped inside.

Step # 03: Setting Your Snare:

When you have properly anchored your snare, push the stick being used as a support deep in the ground. Adjust the height according to the body size of the targeted animal. For instance, if you are setting the trap to catch an opossum then keep the loop one inch higher the ground. It will provide you with the perfect height to capture the animal.

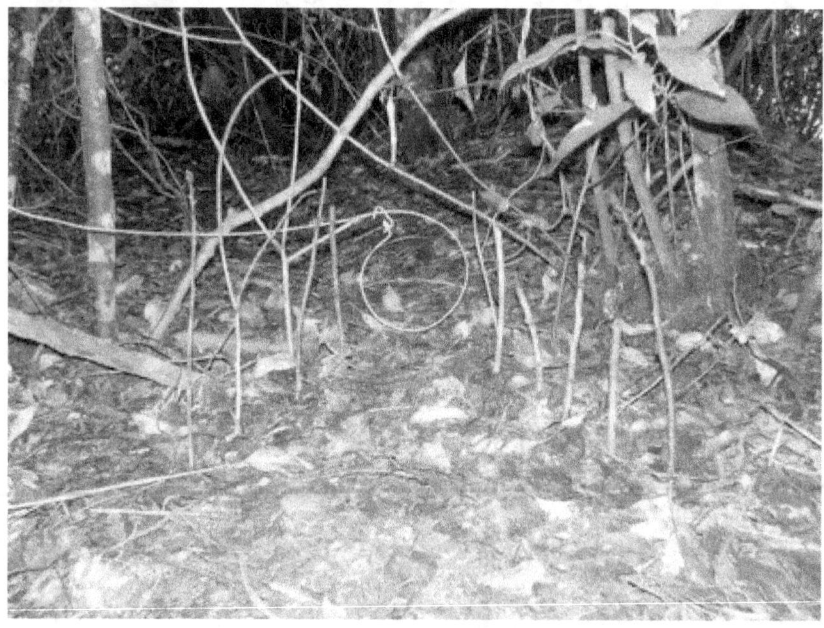

http://cdn.instructables.com/FON/o0OY/I0YGCTXJ/FONo0OYI0YGC-TXJ.MEDIUM.jpg

If you are planning to catch some other animals then this table will help you in setting the snare;

Fox – Height = 6 to 8 inches, Loop = 6 to 8 inches

Coyote – Height = 10 to 12 inches, Loop = 9 to 12 inches

Bobcat – Height = 10 to 12 inches, Loop = 7 to 8 inches

Beaver – Height = 3 inches, Loop = 10 to 12 inches

Raccoon – Height = 3 to 4 inches, Loop = 8 to 9 inches

You can also place some sticks and twigs around the immediate area of the loop and make a fence to guide the targeted animal directly into the loop. It will help you in catching the prey easily.

Step # 04: Checking Your Traps:

It is a good idea to set multiple snares at one location. It will confuse the animal and he will eventually be caught in one of the snares in his struggle to get out of the loops. You need to check all of your snares after every 24 hours. This routine is required by law for all the lands that allow you snaring on them.

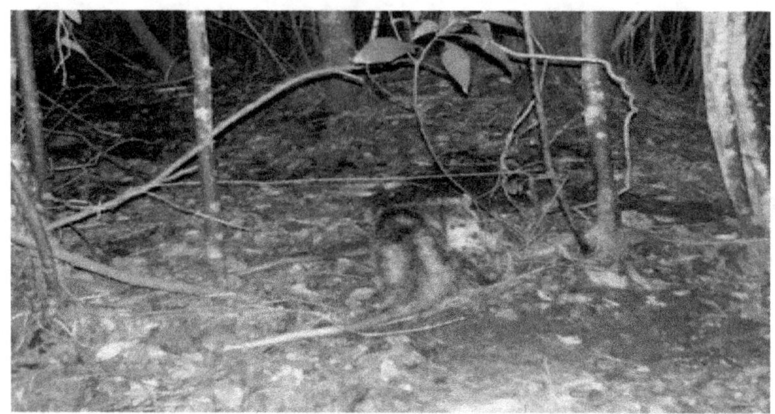

http://cdn.instructables.com/F54/X06Y/I12KHZBL/F54X06Y-I12KHZBL.MEDIUM.jpg

Animals trapped die immediately as the one way lock slides down and the cable gets tighten around their necks. This either quickly breaks their necks or cuts off the blood circulation. You get a quick, bloodless dispatch either way. This is a quick method of hunting and catching your preys without much ado. Snares provide you with fresh, clean catch that you can harvest for meat and fur readily.

Note: It is important to respect all of the animals either dead or alive. If you have caught a prey through a snare then it is your ethical duty to use all parts of the captured animals. For instance, if you have trapped an opossum then preserve its skull and fur and sell them to other crafters. Remember that every part of an animal has its good uses and it is your duty, as a human, to respectfully capture the animals and use every part of the prey.

Chapter 03: Bird Catching Traps and Snares

Snare and traps with loops are a common method of catching birds in the wilderness. A large number of shapes, kinds, sizes and designs of snares and traps are used to hunt birds. Here, we are discussing some of them that can help you hunt whenever you get into a situation to do so;

Bird Catching Snare # 01: Typical Coat Hanger Bird Snare:

A primitive bird trap can be made from a regular coat hanger. It is very easy to make and very effective in capturing the birds. Since all species of birds are edible therefore it is important to make bird traps as you eat them without any kind of endangerment.

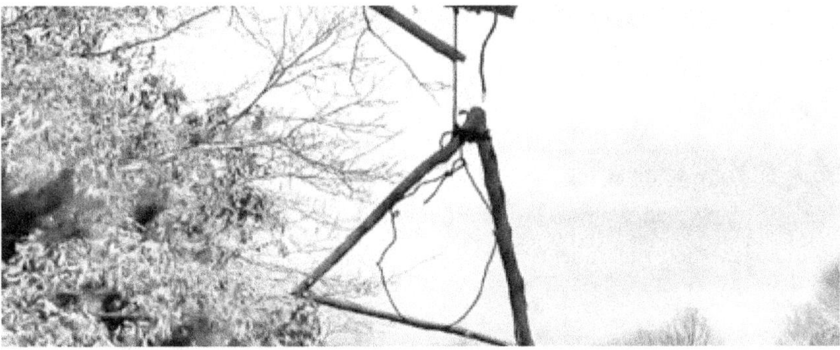

https://www.survivalschool.us/wp-content/uploads/coat-hanger-bird-snare-669x272.png

You can easily make this trap without any tools within a few minutes. The required materials include some woods and a piece of rope. You can also use a regular coat hanger. If you are making it with loose sticks then tie them together to make a V shape. Then add a pedestal stick to go into the V shape.

After shaping the V properly, simply add your snare in this frame. Snare is an effective tool to catch any kind of bird that passes through it. On their main loops, snares have one way locking system. It slides down on a small touch and gets tightened around the neck of the bird. A swivel is added at the end of the cable so the captured bird can move around freely without twisting and thus breaking the cable.

It is a good idea to set multiple snares to catch birds at one location. It will confuse the birds and they will eventually be caught in one of the snares in their struggle to get out of the loops. You need to regularly check your snare to take out the captured birds as hanging dead birds will drive other birds away from that location.

Now you know to make the typical bird snare, you must know the methods of setting and using them as well. Two main methods are mainly used for this purpose i.e. Takiri method and Tahei (taeka) method. Let's read the details together;

Birds Catching Snare # 02: Takiri Method:

A single snare is set on the perch in this method. Feet of the birds are caught in the snares as they sit on them. There are three kinds of snares used under this method;

Mutu Snare:

It is used both on the ground and above in the trees to capture birds. It is made from a single piece of wood. It can take two shapes of either L or T. A loop is draped over the mutu. When a bird lands on the perch, the loop is tugged and the bird is trapped inside.

Tumu Snare:

In it, a small branch is divided into two small branches. These branches are tied at the end then. Snare is laid over these branches. The loop is pulled when a bird lands on it and the prey is captured.

Pewa Snare:

It is used in the similar manner as the previous two snares. The only difference is that it has a strut bracing the upright and the perch which is lashed on it horizontally. Nectar bearing flowers and ripe berries are often tied on loop to bait and trap more birds.

Birds Catching Snare # 03: Tahei (taeka) Method:

Under this method, the snare is kept unattended. And multiple snares are used to capture the birds. They are all tied with slipknots on a single rope and tied horizontally in between branches. The snares are placed near the perch. The birds sit on the perch and get trapped in the snores and killed.

The tree being used to tie the horizontal rope is called taumatua, rakau taeke or rakau tahei. If the snares are set near water then they are called wai taheke or wai tahei.

These snares are usually kept unattended but they are visited once or twice a day as well. It is pertinent to take out the dead birds and reset the snares to catch the new ones. However, you cannot catch kaka with these unattended snares as they can cut down the loop and get free from the trap.

Chapter 04: Catch Reptiles, Snakes and Amphibians

While wandering out in the wild, the snakes, amphibians and reptiles all make a good meal for you. So, you must try to catch them as your dinner meal. It may sound difficult for you to catch them but in reality, it is not that difficult. All you need to know are a few tricks and gather the required material. And you can easily make traps such as snares and wire mesh traps to harvest the wild meal. Here we are discussing a few traps to make in detail. Let's read together!

Method # 01: Catching Snakes, Amphibians and Reptiles with a Snare:

If you want to capture a snake, reptile or an amphibian then this snare is a very easy and safe way to catch some of them especially Gopher snakes and King snakes. Materials that you are going to need to make a simple snare include items such as a nut, a bolt, metal washer, PVC pipe, and rope.

http://cdn.instructables.com/FI3/C75J/IB8PYMSY/FI3C75JIB8PYMSY.MEDI-UM.jpg

Take a PVC pipe of about 4 to 6 foot long. Fold the rope in half and pass it through the pipe down the length. Thread both ends of the rope through the washer and knot it down.

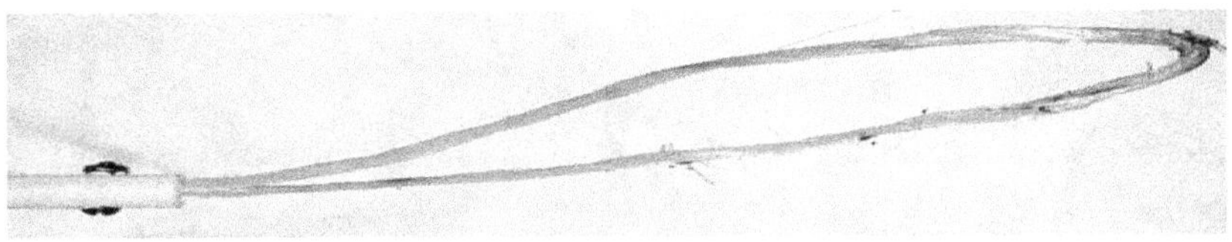

http://cdn.instructables.com/FSV/HZPU/IB8PYMT6/
FSVHZPUIB8PYMT6.LARGE.jpg

Knotting the rope through the washer prevents it getting loose and also provides you with a handle. Now insert a bolt through the PVC pipe one inch from where the loop is heading out. Screw the net. It helps in keeping the loop out of the PVC pipe otherwise you would have to take it out every time.

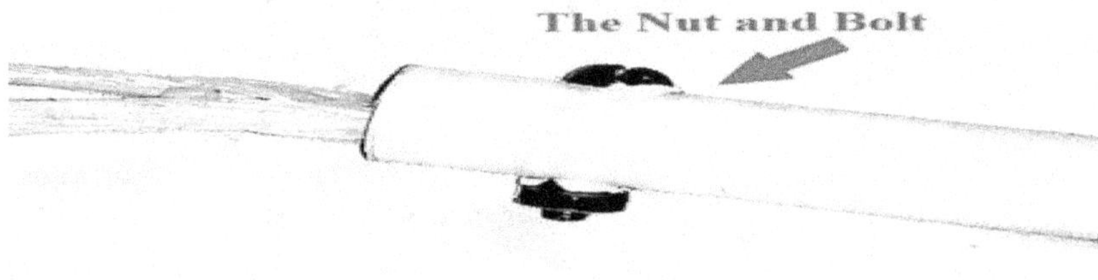

http://cdn.instructables.com/FXX/NLJV/IB8PYMV8/
FXXNLJVIB8PYMV8.MEDIUM.jpg

Now your simple snare is ready and you can use it to capture snakes, reptiles and amphibians in the wild. Use it the same way as you use one to catch dogs in your locality. You need to stay careful and slow while slipping the loop around the neck of the targeted reptile or amphibian. When slipped down, tighten the washer to grip the animal inside the snare loop.

Method # 02: Catching Reptiles, Snakes and Amphibians with Live Catch Trap:

To make a small trap to catch the prey alive is also very easy in the wild. All you need is to gather the materials such as empty steel can. It must be of the size of the targeted animal. For example, if you are planning to catch small lizards then a regular coffee can will work out perfectly.

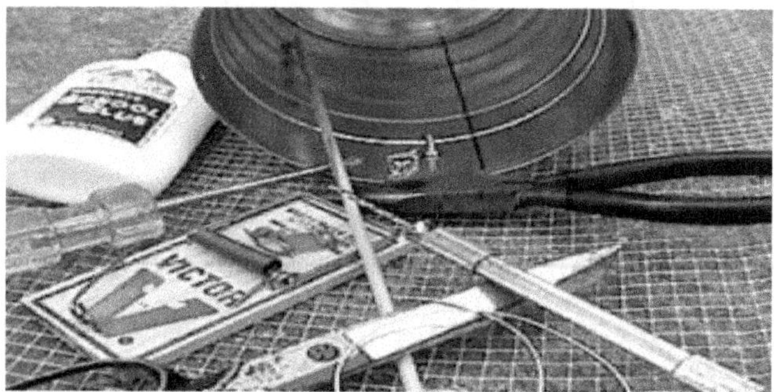

http://cdn.instructables.com/FVD/XX3S/3APEZ439MFF/
FVDXX3S3APEZ439MFF.MEDIUM.jpg

Now you need to mound a mouse trap at the open end of the can. If you don't have a mouse trap in the wild you can use the hooks and wires mesh of anything available in your surroundings to make it like a mouse trap. Keep the mechanism same.

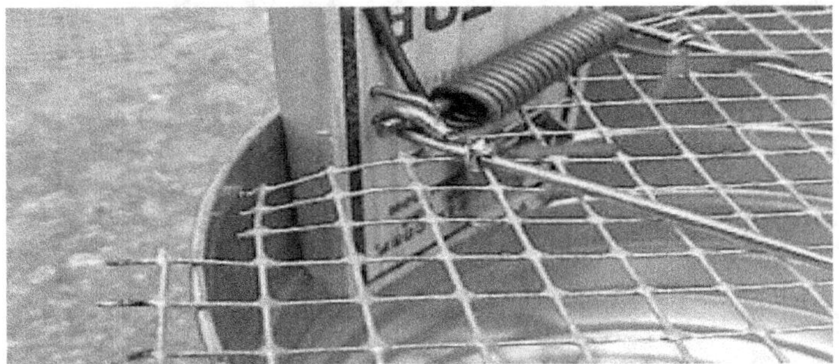

http://cdn.instructables.com/FWP/745V/F8RPG9S3/FWP745VF8RPG9S3.MEDIUM.jpg

Now add a piece of strong wires mesh in the mouse trap and also insert a trigger in the mechanism. This will the wires mesh to get down and close the mouth of the can when the targeted animal will get into the can. Also place some baits inside the can to catch your dinner meal earlier.

Method # 03: Catching Snakes, Reptiles and Amphibians with a Pit Fall Trap:

This is another efficient method of catching live prey for to harvest on the wild meal. This is a very commonly used method. However, a little modification is made by channeling the targeted animal to drop directly inside the hole. This makes the catch easier. You are not going to need much material and technical skills to build this trap as well.

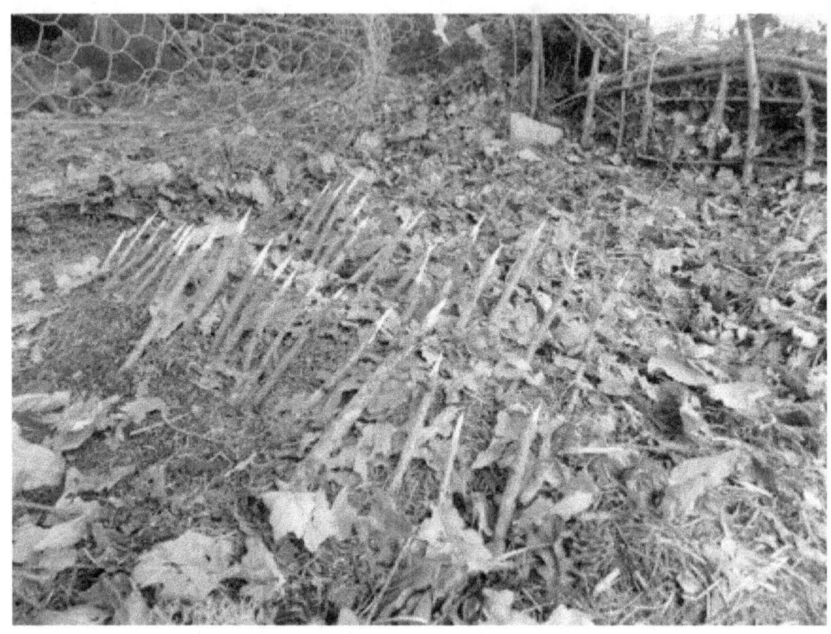

http://cdn.instructables.com/FN6/VTZF/HF23XC3R/FN6VTZFHF23X-C3R.MEDIUM.jpg

First of all, you need to gather many small sticks from around the wild. Make their edges sharper with the help of a blade or a knife. Dig one end of the spikes deep in the ground. Keep their angles a little tilted towards the direction of where you are suppose to dig the hole. Now dig the hole.

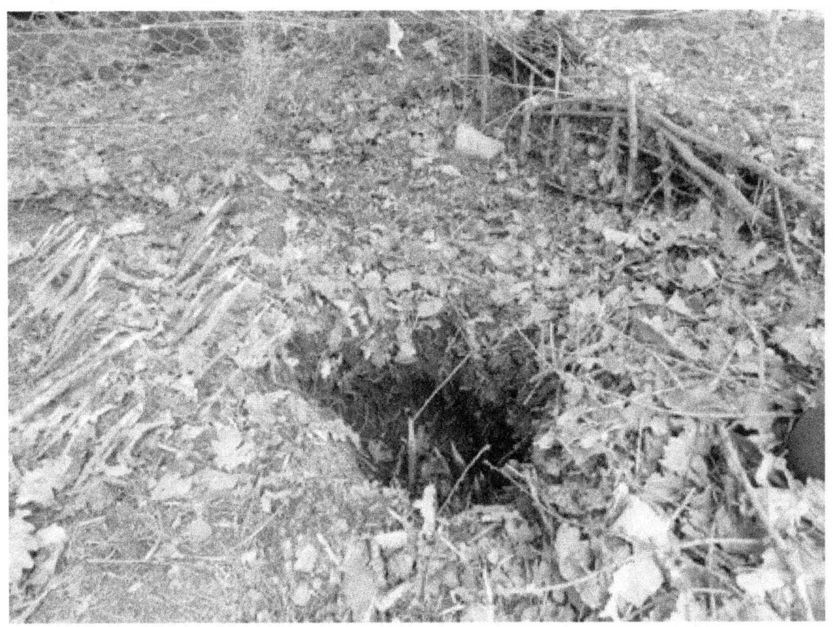

http://cdn.instructables.com/FRP/IO3Q/HF23XC3O/FRPIO3QHF23X-C3O.MEDIUM.jpg

Dig the hole according to the size of the animal that you are planning to catch through this trick. It is pertinent to dig the hole deeper so that the fallen animal does not succeed in getting out of the trap. Another modification that you can make in here is adding spikes at the base of the hole as well. Now spread around all the dry leaves, sticks and twigs to make the trap look a part of the natural landscape. Keep visiting the trap regularly to take out the prey.

Chapter 05: Primitive Fishing Methods

If you are in a wilderness survival scenario and very hungry then fish is the easiest prey for you to catch to get a good deal of meat and protein. If you have a little fishing gear in your survival kit then it's a Yorker! They are many other methods to go fishing in such a scenario as well such as;

Primitive Fishing Method # 01: Hand Fishing:

You can simply go hand fishing your dinner prey. This is the most primitive type of fishing. You actually have to grab a fish with your bare hands from its watery lair. Many names have been given to this activity depending on the geography such as stumping, fish tickling, grabbling, gurgling, cat fisting, hogging, graveling, and noodling.

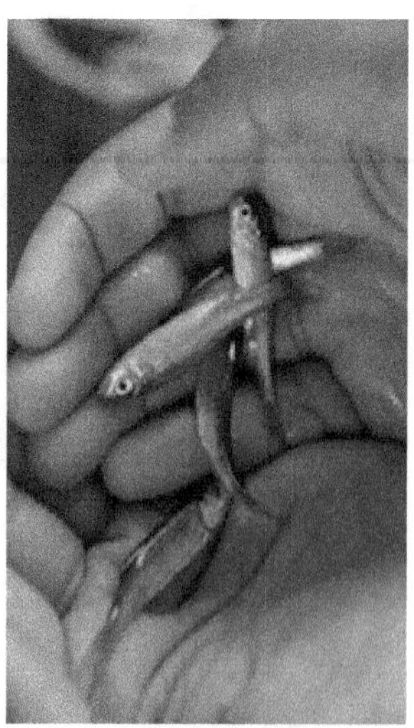

http://images.freeimages.com/images/thumbs/5be/fish-1333105.jpg

However, you cannot get bigger fish with this trick as easily but you will definitely get enough fish for the dinner ahead. You can also wear gloves if you have fear of the murky water.

Primitive Fishing Method # 02: Fishing by Gill Nets:

Most commonly used method is to go fishing with gill nets. The fish get caught in it as soon as they try to pass through the holes of the net.

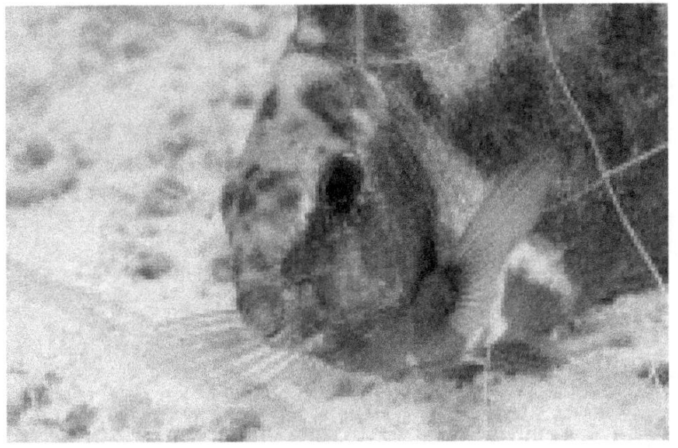

http://i.istockimg.com/file_thumbview_approve/23228764/3/stock-photo-23228764-fish-trapped-in-gill-net.jpg

The gill nets have been proven to be very successful in catching fish however they act as the best tool for during the migration periods.

Primitive Fishing Method # 03: Fishing with a Fish Spear:

Become a real hunter and use a fish spear to catch fish if you don't find any other thing to go fishing. You can easily make a spear from the wood branches lying around in the wild. You must keep a good eye on the fish to hunt it at the exact time to be able to catch it otherwise the slippery creature is going to give big headaches as fishing with a spear requires a lot of patience.

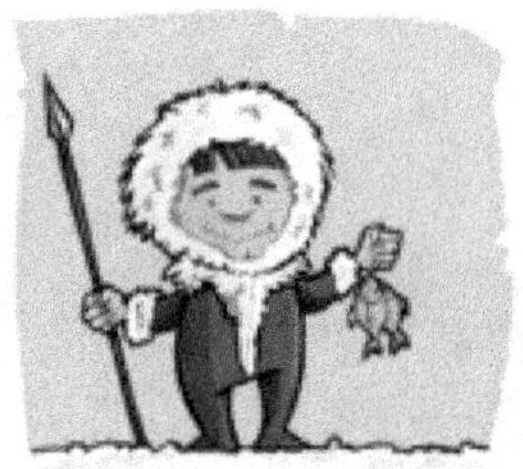

http://i.istockimg.com/file_thumbview_approve/8453359/3/stock-illustration-8453359-eskimo-fisherman.jpg

Spearing the fish is not always successful as it is not easy to defeat the slender profile or pierce the slippery scales of the fish every time. But it is a worthwhile activity to survive in the wild. You must give it a try.

Primitive Fishing Method # 04: Fishing with a Cage Fish Trap:

After a number of unsuccessful attempts at fishing with a spear you can collect some more of them and shape them in a cage fish trap. This is very effective in catching the fish.

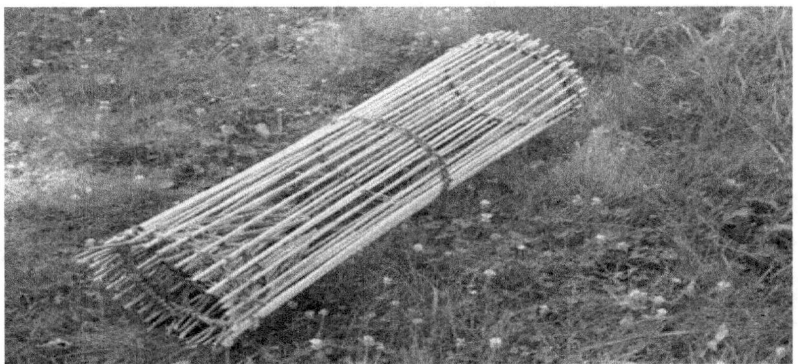

http://www.outdoorlife.com/sites/outdoorlife.com/files/styles/photo-gallery/
public/import/BlogPost/embed/fishtrap6.jpg?itok=qAoq4mfp

First of all, collect the materials. You will need some tree shoots or dowels, a lengthy flexible vine and a knife. Cut all of the tree shoots or dowels in equal lengths. Take the flexible vine and start knitting it through the tree shoots or dowels.

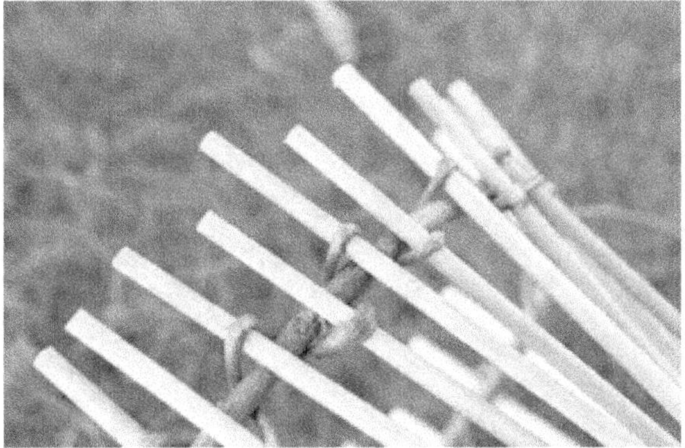

http://www.outdoorlife.com/sites/outdoorlife.com/files/styles/photo-gallery/
public/import/BlogPost/embed/fishtrap2.jpg?itok=D7GxfSau

Knit the flexible vine at both ends of the fish cage and also in the middle. It will strengthen the cage. When you finish the cage then plug one end of it with the help of smaller tree shoots or dowels.

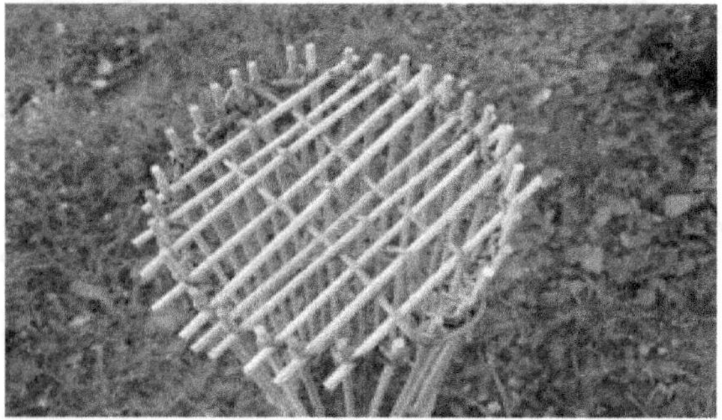

http://www.outdoorlife.com/sites/outdoorlife.com/files/styles/photo-gallery/
public/import/BlogPost/embed/fishtrap4.jpg?itok=9u81B-9c

After plugging the fish cage from one end, it is the time to add a funnel type structure inside the open end of the cage. This will let the fish enter the cage but they will not be able to get of it.

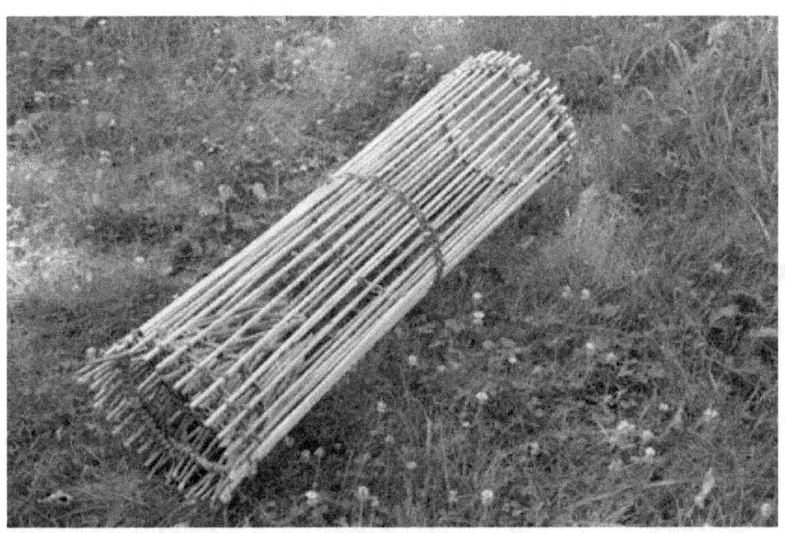

http://www.outdoorlife.com/sites/outdoorlife.com/files/styles/photo-gallery/
public/import/BlogPost/embed/fishtrap6.jpg?itok=qAoq4mfp

Now that your fish cage is ready, you can go fishing now. Simply tie a strong flexible vine at one end of the cage so that you can pull it out of water easily after the fish is caught inside. You can also place baits inside it to capture more prey in less time. Also it is important to place the fish cage in a place inside the water where there is abundance of fish.

Primitive Fishing Method # 05: Fishing with a Fish Funnel Trap:

Another effective method to fish while trying to survive in the wilderness is to make a fish funnel trap with the help of an empty soda bottle. It is very effective method and also the trap is made up easily without much ado. First you need to gather the required materials i.e. an empty soda bottle, a sharp knife, a few feet of string or flexible vine and a few pieces of meat or any other bait.

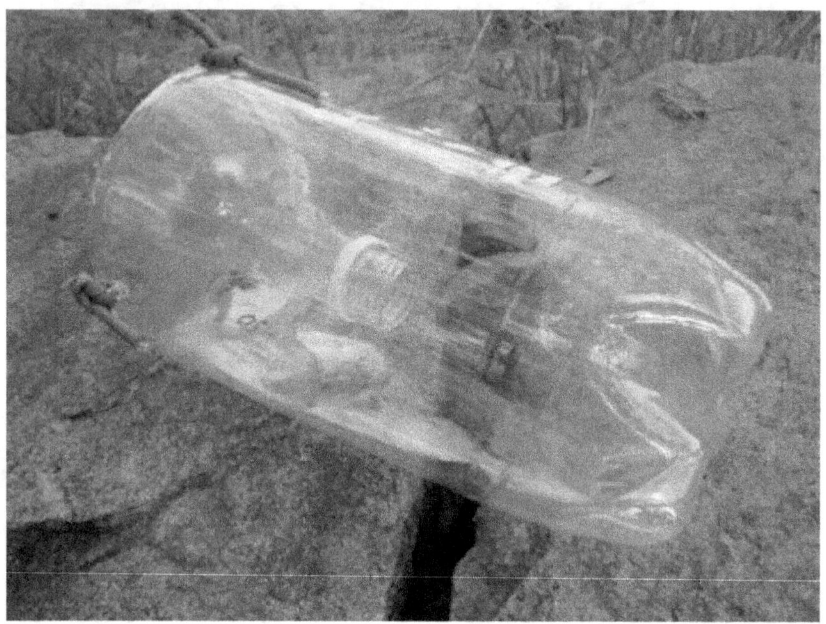

http://www.outdoorlife.com/sites/outdoorlife.com/files/styles/photo-gallery/
public/import/BlogPost/embed/P1011739.jpg?itok=AxWrMlC8

Simply cut the upper half of the bottle and place it inside the lower portion in the inverted direction. This will allow the fish to go inside the bottle but they won't be able to figure out the way out of the trap. Place in the bait or a few pieces of meat and put the bottle in the water at a place where there is abundance of fish. Keep the flexible vine or the string in your hand or tie with a nearby solid thing or a tree.

Chapter 06: Protect Meat from Critters:

If you are stuck somewhere in the wilderness or just want to feed your family with a flavorful, wholesome and all-natural food then harvesting your own game food is a good technique for you to satisfy the craving.

Before the Hunt:

Before going on the hunt, unless you are stuck in some wilderness and you don't have your survival kit with you, keep the following items with you i.e. canvas or tarps, clean rags, wipes or paper towels, game bags and saw, sharp hunting knife, disposable or rubber gloves and a rope. Black pepper and cheesecloth are optional items for you to take with you on the hunt.

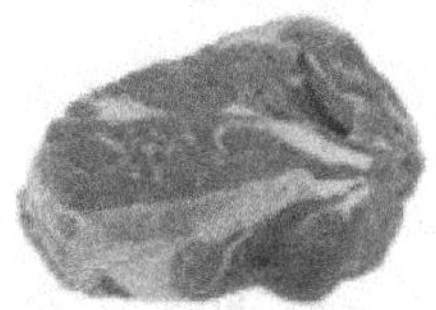

http://images.freeimages.com/images/thumbs/f00/meat-1324654.jpg

During the Hunt:

Choose the right type of the trap for the kind of animal you are striving to hunt in the wilderness. If you are shooting the animal then strive for a clean shot because the meat can get contaminated with the intestinal contents if you shot the body with a gut shot.

After the Hunt:

It is a fair possibility that you cannot completely finish the hunt. The remaining meat is to be secured in a manner that it does not age that fast and also you need to keep it safe from the critters such as mice, lemmings, voles, rats, chipmunks, and many others. Here we are discussing the food protection techniques in the wild, let's read together;

Meat Protection Techniques:

There a number of techniques through which you can protect your meat from the critters. Here, we are looking at some of the most adopted ones; they are easy and effective;

Meat Protection Technique # 01: Do Not Camp Where You Cook:

Never ever camp where you cook your food. Keep a distance of at least a few hundred yards from your camp when you cook the meat. Also prefer an area with a lot of air so the scent of the cooking meat is dispersed and critters and other animals do not get attracted by it.

Meat Protection Technique # 02: Do Not Keep Scented Items with the Meat:

Another technique to keep the critters away from the meat is not to keep any scented items with it. These items include things such as sweet smelling toothpastes, deodorants, slabs of bacon, and fresh T-bone steaks. All of these items will attract the critters which you obviously do not want to happen.

Meat Protection Technique # 03: Burn down the Trash:

It is also a good method to burn down the trash o regular basis. This reduces the scents especially if the trash contains bones and leftovers of meat in it. Rodents and critters are highly attracted to such items. And this can lead them to the meat that you have saved for your coming day food.

Meat Protection Technique # 04: Do Not Travel and Camp Near Food Sources of Other Animals:

It is always better not to travel and camps near the food sources and trails of other animals. These places stay crowded with the animals and they can easily attract towards your saved meat and camp as well. This can be dangerous for you so it is good to stay away from the trails and food sources of other animals.

Meat Protection Technique # 05: Tuck the Remaining Meat in Rocks:

If you happen to be in an area with a lot of rocks then you have a fair chance of finding a natural protection for the meat. You can easily find a nook in these rocks where you can tuck in the meat. You can also scramble up a piece of rock and put the meat in the ledge.

Meat Protection Technique # 06: Use Canisters:

If you have found some kind of canisters made up of carbon fiber or plastic then it becomes very easy for you to protect your meat both from aging and the critters.

Meat Protection Technique # 07: Sleep with Your Food:

If there is no other method to protect the meat from the rodents and critters then you have to sleep with it. Any animal trying to reach your food and the meat will make some kind of noise in the process and this can wake you up. Thus you will be there to protect the meat from them.

Conclusion

In a survival situation, take care of the most important needs first. These needs are prioritized according to the actual scenario and situation. The most important thing to find in the wild is a safe source of food that you can eat without any kind of endangerment. Unless you have complete or extensive knowledge about the fauna and flora of the area you happen to be at the time and you are much adaptive to hunting and trapping, you are not going to fulfill your basic needs of 1500 calories a day.

It is not easy to survive in the wild on your own but it is not impossible as well. Remember that 95% of the wilderness emergency situations are resolved in the first 72 hours of getting into the situation either by self extraction or outside rescue.

All you need is to have an extensive knowledge of the flora and fauna and some of the hunting and trapping techniques to capture the important sources of food abundant in protein and fat such as fish, amphibians and reptiles etc.

Building Your Own Shelter That Will Stand up a Storm

Introduction

Shelters are necessary to provide protection against the harsh weathers in the wild. Also, they serve as a first defense against the enemies as you can hide inside and wait for the right moment to attack, if necessary. Picking up a location for your campsite is a critical decision not only for the security purposes but self-reliance opportunities as well.

There are many methods and techniques through which you can build shelters robust enough to stand a storm. Camouflaging your shelter is pertinent. It not only provides you protection from the wild animals but also helps you hide your location from the unfriendly strangers.

You can also build shelters in snow. They are made to create an insulating environment for your survival under harsh and cold weather conditions. These shelters can maintain a constant temperature of 36 degrees centigrade. Lighting a tea candle take it up to 40 degrees inside.

You can build your temporary accommodation on a mountain too. But you must consider the risk factors and self-reliance opportunities before constructing one.

Chapter 01: Tips to Select a Mountain to Build Your Shelter

Picking up a location for your campsite is a critical decision not only for the security purposes but self-reliance opportunities as well. Mountains are preferred over other sites because natural water resources are readily available there and also, more possibilities of self-defense are available. Here, we are discussing a few important tips to select a mountain to build your shelter. Let's read together;

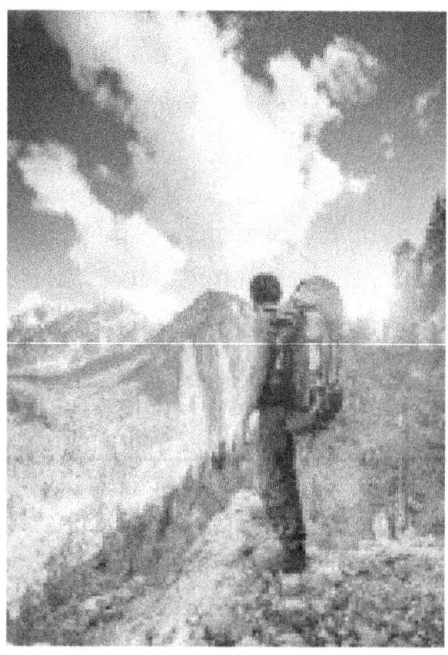

http://i.istockimg.com/file_thumbview_approve/75505359/3/stock-photo-75505359-young-man-traveler-with-backpack-relaxing-outdoor.jpg

Location Distance to the Mountain:

There are two primary aspects of your campsite at the mountain in figuring out the location distance:

1. The entire traveling distance of the campsite

2. The distance between your campsite and the first dense population

Keeping traveling distance of your campsite location as short as possible is pertinent. The further you will take to reach your campsite location from your current home, the more problems you are going to face in the way such as roadblock set ups within hours.

If you are walking to your campsite at the mountain from your current home, then it must be less than a five days distance. One day travel must not exceed 12 miles. It means that the overall distance from the location of the campsite at the mountain must not more than sixty miles away from your current home.

If you are driving to your campsite at the mountain from your current home, then it must not be farther than where one tank of fuel can take you. Getting long-term reliable fuel storage is pertinent if you are planning to go farther than one fuel tank distance. No matter how much fuel you store, it is never advisable to set your campsite farther than a fuel tank distance from your current home.

The second aspect in figuring out the location distance of your campsite at the mountain is its proximity to high-density population.

Your checklist must include:

- Figuring out the distance to check if you can travel between your current home and the desired campsite location within five days on the walk and within a fuel tank while driving.

- Checking if the campsite you want on the mountain is present at a fair distance from the nearest high-density population.

Water Availability at the Mountain:

It is ideal to have a natural water source near your campsite on the mountain. It is not possible to survive without water for quite a long time, therefore, having access to natural water resources like a stream, river, lake, or pond at such sites is pertinent.

Otherwise, you need to have self-replenishing massive water storage system. It consists of rainwater storage systems and large storage tanks.

Abundant water can go way beyond just hydrating you. You can use it for sanitation. You can harness energy through a consistent power generation system on it as well.

You can quickly set-up a hydro-power generation system if you have running water nearby your campsite on the mountain that falls a slope at a decent speed.

Your check list must include:

- What are the nearby fresh water resources at the campsite location on the mountain?

- How reliable are those resources?

- How far are they exactly from the campsite?

- Bonus point: if the water supply is high enough to have kinetic energy?

Securing and Concealing Your Mountain:

After checking the distance of your campsite location from the high-density population, securing and hiding it is pertinent. Unfriendly people may locate you if you are not careful enough. You have found the site, so there is a fair chance for other people to discover it too.

Find locations that are not near to the mountain pass or traveling paths. People go on these routes more often. They can locate you and your campsite. Find locations that are not near to the mountain pass or traveling paths. People travel on these paths more often. They can easily locate you and your campsite.

After finding one good location, you need to conceal your tent, RV, shelter or cabin on it. A camouflaged location is not easy to find. Also, wanderers cannot see you from a distance.

Also, check if the smoke and scent, when you heat or cook, will attract people to your location or not. It is ideal to contain your fire during the daytime and light it at night only. It will hide the smoke.

Another important thing is to check that how many people are using the natural water resource that you have located for your use. Too many people coming there is not okay for your campsite.

Your checklist must include:

- How can you camouflage your location and tent?

- If people can detect smoke and scent of your cooking and heating from a fair distance?

- How much populated is the nearby natural water resource?

Self-Reliance Opportunities at Your Mountain:

We have discussed hydro-power generation earlier. If you are camping in an area with a lot of sunlight, then you can check out the solar power generating ideas as well.

Also, test the food-producing potential of soil around your campsite. If the mountain is all rocks and no soil then growing a vegetable garden, there is going to be a challenge for you.

You will also need abundant firewood around your campsite. Therefore, too much rocky area with no trees does not suit you.

You may also plan to raise some livestock on the location for food. Check if there is enough grass to feed them. You may also need to grow food to support your chickens.

Your checklist must include:

- Is there enough sunlight to install a solar panel for power generation?

- What is the food-producing potential of the soil around your campsite?

- Does the area contain abundant firewood?

- Can you raise livestock at the campsite or not?

Chapter 02: Half-cave and Fallen Tree Shelter

Shelters are necessary to provide protection against the harsh weathers in the wild. Also, they serve as a first defense against the enemies as you can hide inside and wait for the right moment to attack, if necessary.

There are many methods and techniques through which you can build shelters robust enough to stand a storm. In this chapter, we are discussing two primitive types of such accommodations i.e. half-cave and fallen tree shelter. You can build on your own to fight the harsh weathers.

The Half-cave Shelter:

Shelters provide protection from the sun or rain and snow. Therefore, you only need them when the weather starts playing tricks with you. The easiest among all of the temporary shelters out there is the half-cave shelter. It has a lean-to structure. You only need to build a roof and erect walls on the sides.

Building the Roof:

Step # 01: Locating an Overhanging Cliff:

Using an over-hanging cliff for this shelter is optimal as you don't have to do much work. There are many other benefits in using over-hanging cliffs as a roof for your half-cave shelter as well. They are excellent at providing defense from the enemies as well as protection from the harsh weathers.

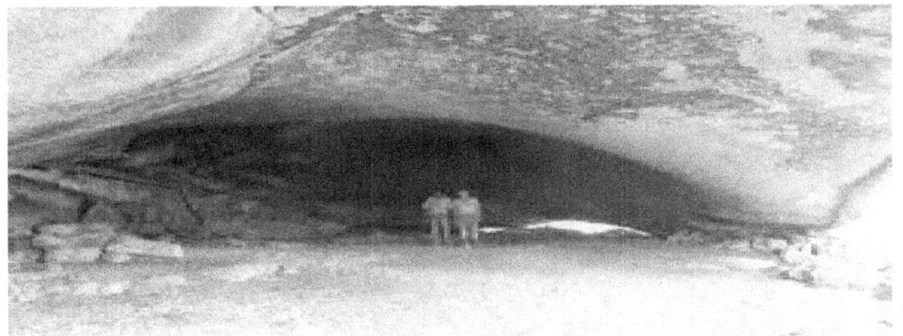

Step # 02: Finding Long Poles or Branches:

If you are unable to locate any over-hanging cliff in the current area, then you must find a pole or a stable branch of eight to ten meters in length. Secure this pole or branch to a sturdy tree at the height of your waistline. It will allow you to sit straight inside.

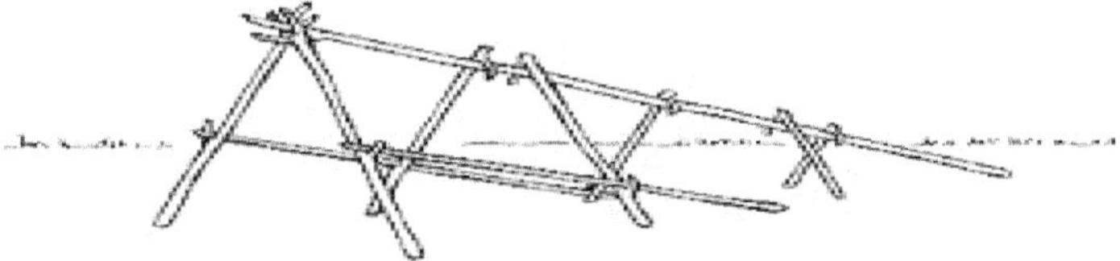

Rest the other end of the pole on the ground. Fix it in there so it does not move or slide with the wind. Add more branches on the sides to strengthen the framework. Now is the turn to build walls.

Building the Walls:

Step # 01: Collecting the Green Boughs:

Gather a few green boughs. The leaves must adhere to them. They will provide you shade from direct sunlight and also, will protect you from drizzling raindrops in the first few days of the build. Torrential rains can enter inside. Once the leaves get dry, put some fresh green boughs on the previous ones.

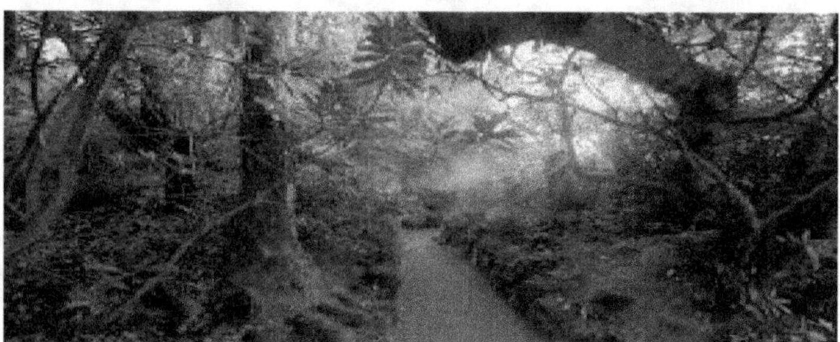

Remember that you can have some uninvited friends on these green branches such as insects and ants. But they are part of the green. You cannot get rid of them all together.

Step # 02: Resting the Green Boughs:

Rest all of the green boughs against the cliff or the pole. It is important to rest all of the boughs on their heads on the ground. Use flexible green branches to thatch the branches to build the basic framework.

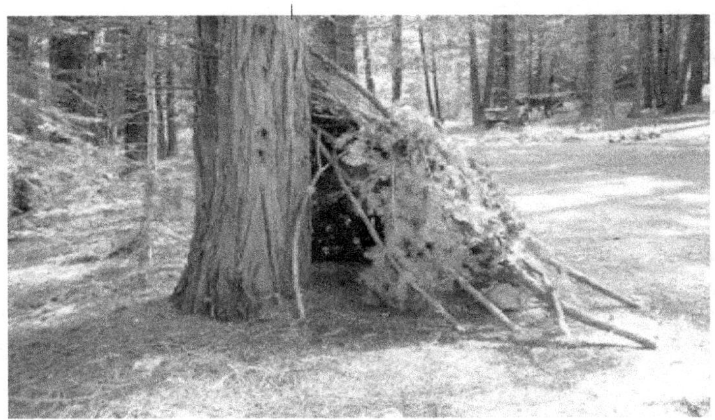

The reason for placing them this way is to steer the water to the ground. Erecting them in straight position will lever the rain drops into the shelter, and you will get no place to sit in there.

Step # 03: Camouflaging the Shelter:

No shelter made out there in the wild is safe. You can make it strong enough to stand the storms but hiding it will provide you protection and safety from both the wild animals and unfriendly passer-bys.

For camouflaging, gather some branches (both green and dried) from your immediate surroundings. Add a layer of the gathered wood on the sides and roof of your temporary accommodation. You can also add a layer of dried leaves or fill them in between the gaps of the branches to match the surroundings.

The Fallen-tree Shelter:

These temporary accommodations use less wood and have an original build. You can create them on a fallen tree by adding branches and poles on the sides to strengthen the framework and then laying layers of green boughs to provide coverage.

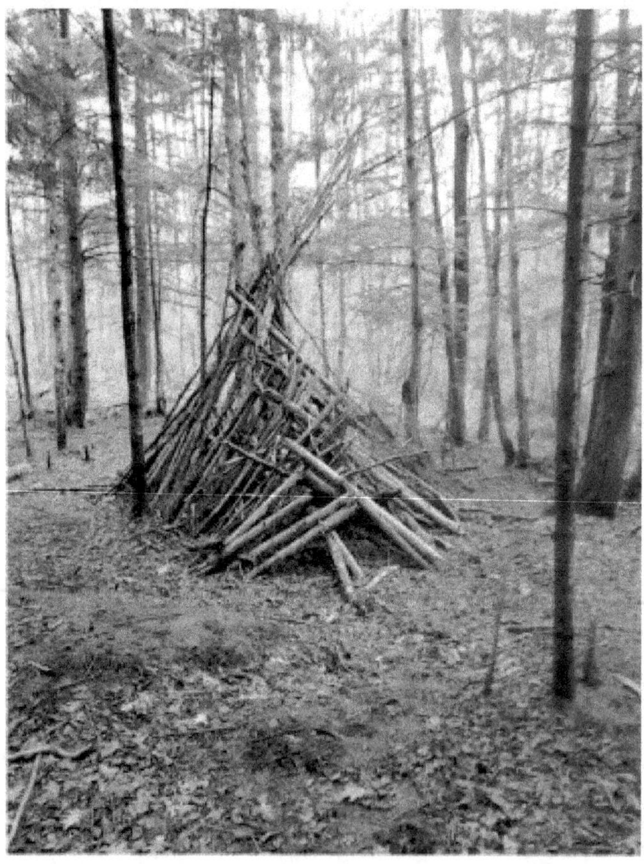

Building the Roof:

Step # 01: Locating a Fallen Tree:

The first step to building this kind of shelter is to find a fallen tree. It must be on the highest and driest ground. It must be robust enough to take the load of branches and high sufficiently to accommodate you under it.

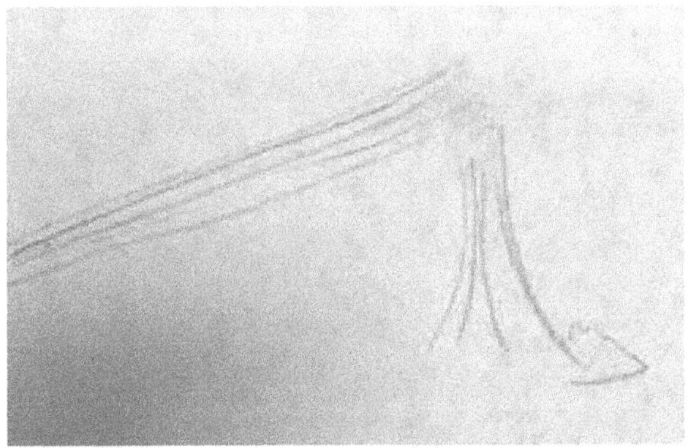

Step # 02: Cutting a Tree:

If you are unable to find a fallen tree in the surroundings, then you can cut if down yourself as well. Cut it partly through the trunk and drop it on the other side. It is pertinent to cut a tree that already has thick green branches. It will reduce the workload for you.

Building the Walls:

Step # 01: Gathering and Cutting Appropriate Boughs:

After you have found or cut a fallen tree, gather some branches. The quantity depends on upon how green is the fallen tree already. Add sturdy branches at a suitable distance from the fallen trunk to strengthen the framework.

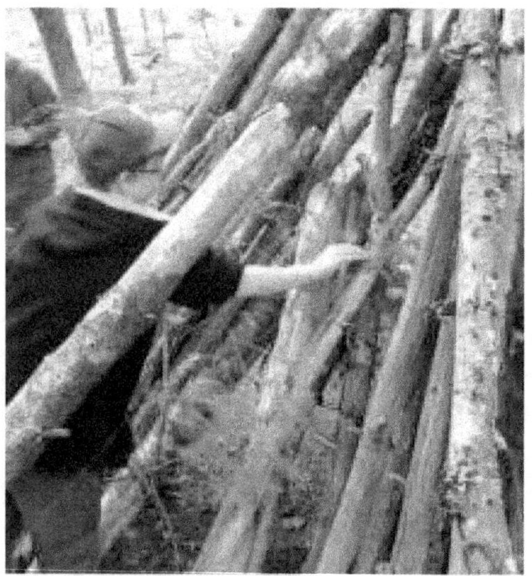

Step # 02: Secure the Branches:

After you have completed the structure, start adding small green branches in it to provide coverage. Place all the branches up-side-down. This position of the branches will steer the water to the ground. Erecting them in straight position will lever the raindrops into the shelter, and you will get no place to sit in there.

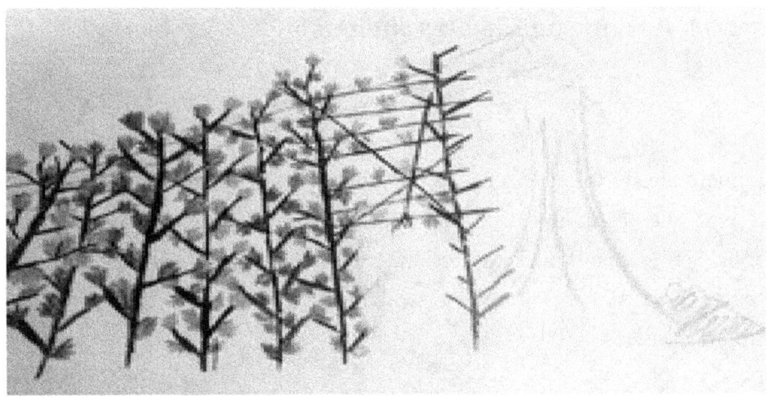

Step # 03: Camouflaging the Shelter:

Camouflaging your shelter is pertinent. It not only provides you protection from the wild animals but also helps you hide your location from the unfriendly strangers. Use branches and leaves from the immediate surroundings for camouflaging.

Chapter 03: A Frame and TeePee Shelters

It is pertinent always to plan before jumping into the process of building a shelter. The first rule of thumb to consider is to estimate the time you are going to spend in it. The Second thing is to check the weather before determining the type of shelter to build. We are discussing two types of primitive shelters for you in this chapter.

Building an A-Frame Shelter:

A-frame shelters are easy to create and provide you ample protection from the sun and rain. You can use them for extended periods. They are also easily camouflaged.

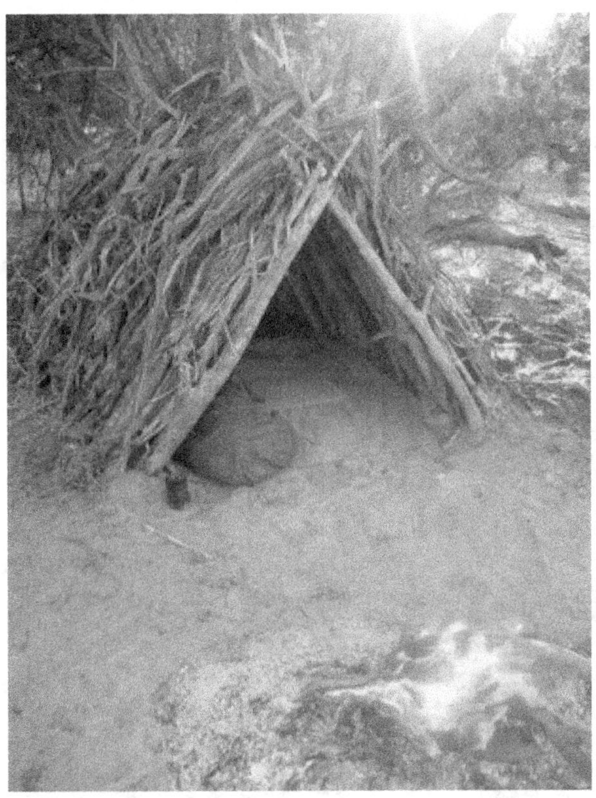

http://cdn.instructables.com/FW0/T4H7/HUDEPJN9/
FW0T4H7HUDEPJN9.MEDIUM.jpg

Step # 01: Finding a Location:

Choose a site to construct the A-frame shelter. It is pertinent to identify the risks before deciding the place. Stay away from the traveling rails. Also, avoid the dense area with thick trees as most of the wild animals like to inhabit in such areas.

Step # 02: Constructing the Frame:

You need one long pole to run it along the top, two small poles to make the arms of the ridgepole, sturdy branches of different sizes to make the ribs, flexible branches or rope to secure the framework and a lot of dry leaves and branches to fill the frame. Gather the wood.

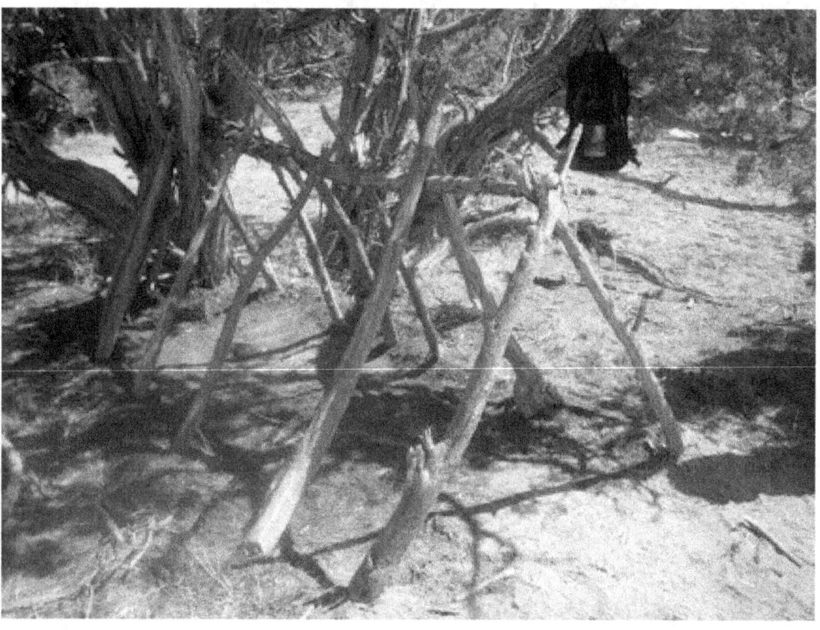

http://cdn.instructables.com/FCW/FGBQ/HUDEPJON/FCWFGBQHUDE-PJON.MEDIUM.jpg

Take the longest among all poles and make it the central beam. If it is not long enough, then tie two branches together. Insert one end of this pole in the ground firmly. Take two small branches and secure them with the hanging end of the pole. Rest these arms on the ground. Add ribs to the framework.

Step # 03: Filling in the Framework:

Gather as many small green and dried branches as much thick you want your temporary house to be. Camouflaging your shelter to its surroundings is pertinent. Therefore, always pick the filling and thatching material from the immediate environment. Gather the material and fill in the gaps of the structure. There must not be any holes left in it. Also, place long green branches on their heads. It will draw the rainwater directly to the ground, and the inside area of your temporary home will not get flooded.

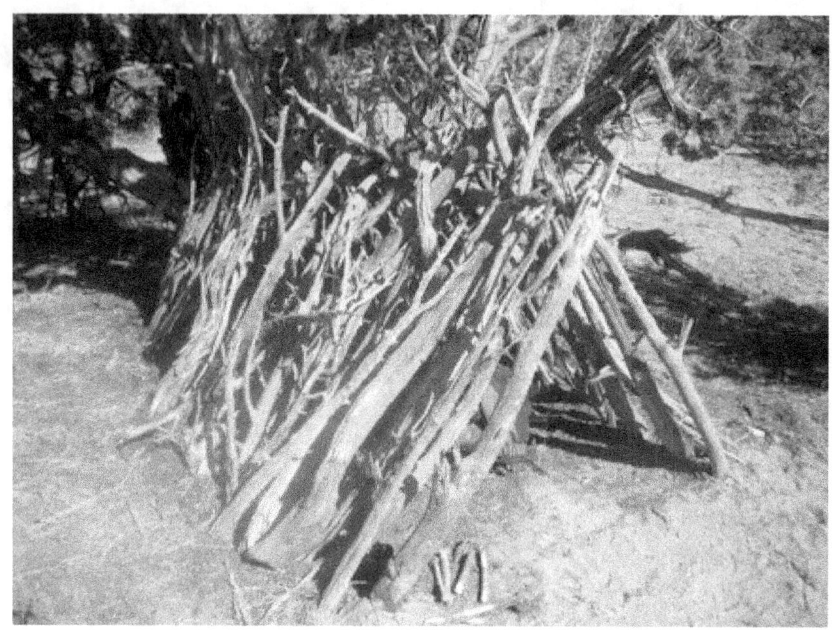

http://cdn.instructables.com/FJE/Q7WW/HUDEPJOE/FJEQ7WWHUDE-PJOE.MEDIUM.jpg

Building a Teepee Shelter:

Teepee shelters are very much like the A-frame shelters, but they provide less inner space than them. And you can make them anywhere. They are portable too.

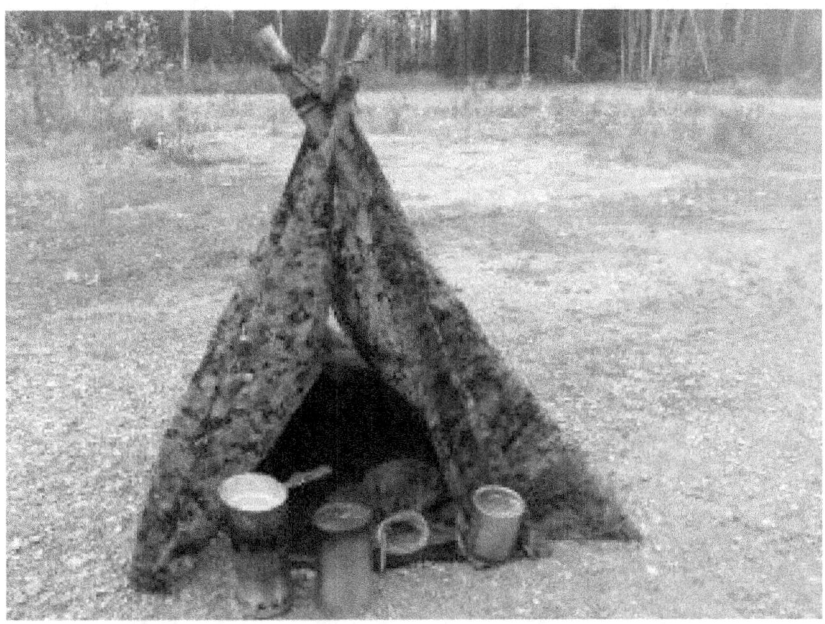

http://cdn.instructables.com/FDL/UP42/GTGCVL9K/FDLUP42GT-GCVL9K.MEDIUM.jpg

Step # 01: Picking up the Sticks:

After selecting a safe and risk-free location, probably near a natural water source, it is the time to gather sticks for your teepee shelter. Collecting right type of sticks for the framework is pertinent. Otherwise, it can result in a total loss both in terms of time and efforts. You need three main poles. One must be taller than your head. The other two must reach your height. The poles must be two to three inches wide, and the must not be broken from anywhere. If any of them is broken then first, lash it firmly before incorporating it into the framework.

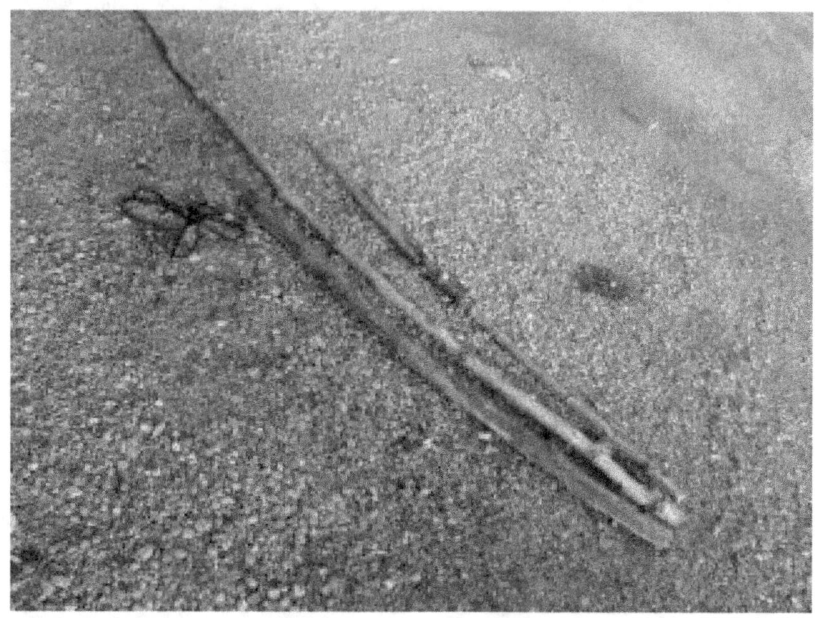

http://cdn.instructables.com/FNG/7KDK/GT9U8OB2/
FNG7KDKGT9U8OB2.MEDIUM.jpg

Step # 02: Lashing the Sticks Together:

Place all three of the sticks on the ground. Balance their tops. Now fasten them together firmly. Using rope or shoe laces for this purpose is ideal. But in the wild, you can also use flexible branches to tie the sticks up. Keep the knots real tight.

Step # 03: Standing the Frame up:

After you have tied them all together tightly, now stand the structure on the ground. Wedge the ends of the poles into the ground firmly. You can also place heaps of mud and small stones around the wedged poles to strengthen the framework.

Spread the arms of the structure and insert them into the ground as well. You do not need to put ribs in the frame. It is a small structure that you are going to use for sitting purposes mostly.

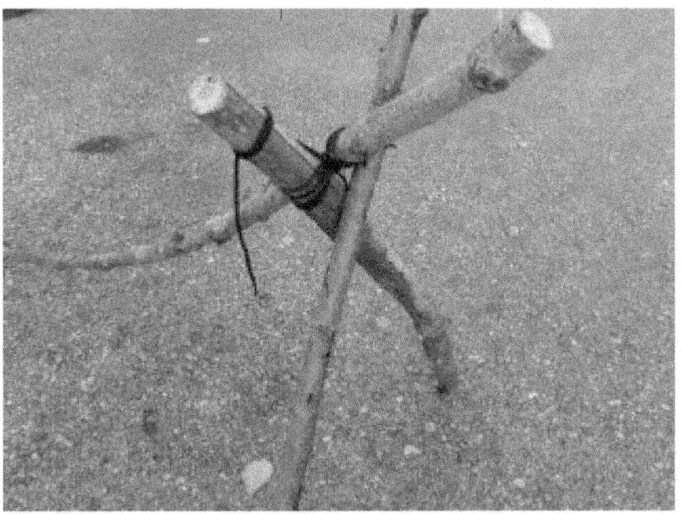

http://cdn.instructables.com/FPJ/8oR2/GT9U8P2Z/ FPJ8oR2GT9U8P2Z.MEDIUM.jpg

Step # 04: Covering the Framework:

After wedging the poles firmly into the ground, you are ready to cover the structure. You can use dry leaves and green branches for this purpose. Also, camouflage your shelter to the surroundings. It is helpful in providing you protection from both the wild animals and unfriendly strangers. As the shelter is all made up of wood, it is pertinent to light the fire outside your temporary accommodation.

Chapter 04: Tips to Build Indian Shelters and Shacks

Native red men of India have developed many designs and styles in temporary shelters. They are being used successfully by them for centuries. However, they come with the defects of ill ventilation and dirtiness. But they are very useful in providing shade and shelter. We are discussing various kinds of Indian shelters and shacks and the tips for building them accurately in the chapter. Let's read together!

Tips for Building Indian Navajo:

Navajo is a teepee shape shelter. Navajo Indian adopted this style in shelters to shed the rain. It is very easy to build and lasts for an extended period.

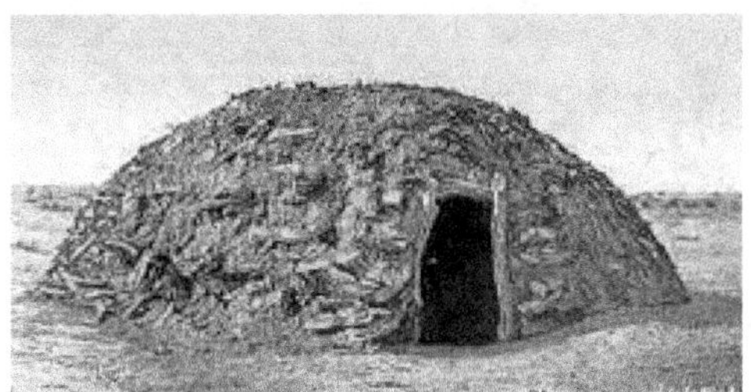

Framework: Its structure includes three forked sticks and other poles and branches. Its framework has the shape of a teepee shelter. Insert three sturdy sticks into the ground nearby in the form of a circle. Interlock the forked sticks together at the top.

Layering: Navajo Indians layer this framework with dirt. But if you are building it in the wild as a survival tool then you must use branches and leaves from the immediate surroundings to fill the structure. It will camouflage your shelter. This camouflaging helps you in hiding in the wild both from the dangerous animals and unfriendly strangers.

Tips for Building Indian Adobe Roof:

Adobe is a mixture of material for building roofs on your shelters. Straw and dirt are mixed and baked into hard bricks to make adobe roofs. Using large stones is also an option here. Yo can place them on the ceiling.

Filling the Roof: You can use sod, rushes, grass, hay, straws, dry or green leaves, and browse and small boughs to cover the poles in the wild.

Slanting the Roof: You can also slant the roof of your shelter instead of keeping it straight. Straight roofs only provide shades from the sun. A slanting roof protects you from almost any kind of climate.

Tips for Building Indian White Men's Walls:

White men keep walls of their shelters perpendicular to each other. It provides more space inside the accommodation than the other styles of temporary accommodations. But the problem here is that you cannot find suitable material to fill these walls in the wild.

Erecting Planting Walls: Therefore, erecting planting walls are more appropriate for building shelters in the wild than in the countryside. Dry leaves and green branches are used to layer these walls which are easier than the vertical ones.

Camouflaging Your Shelter: Also, this kind of walls make it easy for you to hide your refuge in the wild as it's hard to find straightly erected frameworks there. Planting walls make it very much a part of the surroundings in the wild.

Tips for Building Indian Pima Lodge:

It is an amazing style of shelter widely adopted by a majority of the Indians. The amazing quality of Pima lodge lies in adapting to the necessities of the surroundings like getting warm and tight or fresh and airy as per the climate.

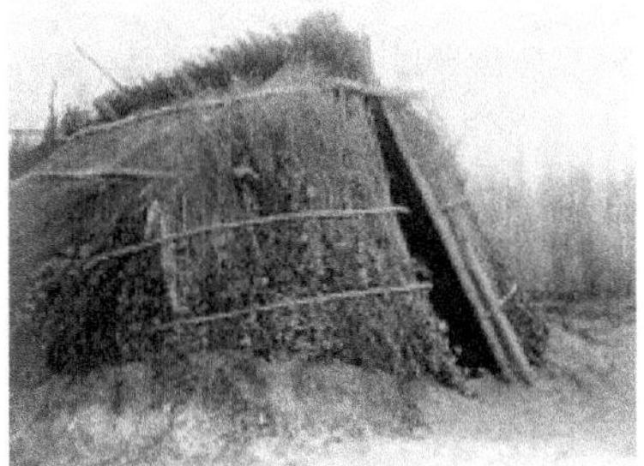

Framework: The structure of Pima lodge is like that of wick-up shelters. However, the sides of this lodge consist of leaning poles instead of the four upright posts. It makes it more adaptable to the wild surroundings. Again, it is helpful in camouflaging.

Tips for Building Indian Chippewa Shack:

Chippewa shacks are a modification of the San Carlos Apache.

Framework: These shacks have a similar dome-shaped frame like San Carlos Apache, but the layering on the structure is entirely different from that of the Apache.

Layering: Chippewa Indians use this kind of shelter mostly. They cover the structure with layers of birch bark. They are kept in place with the help of ropes. However, this practice is not possible in the wild. Therefore, you can use branches, palm leaves, palmetto leaves, straw, hay, and browse to thatch the walls. You can also plaster them with mud.

Tips for Building Indian San Carlos Shack:

San Carlos shack is a dome-shaped framework of small saplings.

Framework: You can find these young branches in the wild quickly. The ends of these branches or poles are sunk in the ground firmly in the form of a circle. You can also repeat the series by making an inner circle of these small saplings as well.

Roof: The free ends of these poles are bent and tied at the top. It gives it the shape of a dome and also provides strength and stability to the structure as the overlapping saplings are interlocked.

Layering: In the countryside, the framework is thatched with overlapping rows of bear-grass. However, in the wild, you can plaster it with mud or fill with dry leaves and green branches.

Tips for Building Indian Apache Hogan:

It is a traditional tent shape Indian shack. It has the particular framework and layering, but the difference is that rank grass instead of birch bark is used for layering this framework. You can also use corn-stalks to thatch the structure in the wild.

Building shelters are inevitable for survival in the wild and on your campsite. Indians have invented and modified several shelters and shacks over the time. However, these temporary accommodations are often ill ventilated and dirty. Both of these defects can be drawn away. You can build Windows in any of these styles by considering the element factors of the surroundings such as the kind of wild animals wandering around and the type of weather you are experiencing at that time. Else, all of these shelters are protective and have an easy built.

Chapter 05: How to build a shelter in snow

Snow shelters are made to create an insulating environment for your survival under harsh and cold weather conditions. These shelters can maintain a constant temperature of 36 degrees centigrade. Lighting a tea candle take it up to 40 degrees inside. It happens because snow is composed of trapped air. You can survive in these temporary accommodations without adequate sleeping material or clothing. Also, you don't need many tools, equipment, and materials to build these snow shelters, and you need only basic knowledge.

Step # 01: Identifying Risks:

It is pertinent to identify all kinds of risks that you can encounter at the location where you intend to build your snow shelter. Do not construct the accommodation at an area that is going to be wiped out by falling trees, falling rocks, avalanche, and landslide or similar.

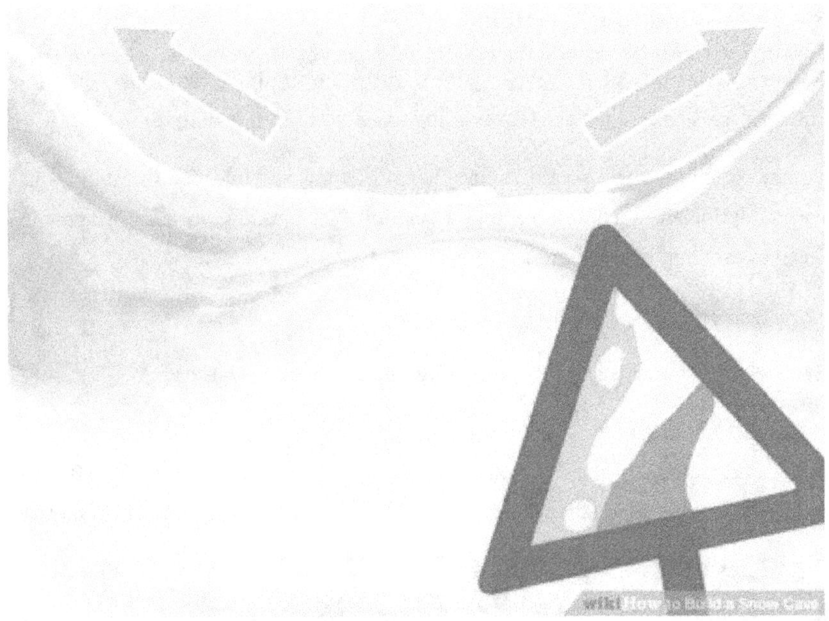

It can be difficult for you to locate your snow shelter if you leave at night or during a storm. It is recommendable to mark it with a bright color flag so you can reach it back. These flags also prevent you walking over the shelter and thus, collapsing it.

It is pertinent to poke a breathing hole in your snow shelter as carbon monoxide, and carbon dioxide can trap inside if you are lightening a candle.

The construction process is tiring, and you can sweat. Therefore, take off the insulating layers of your clothing and wear the waterproof jackets as the process can cover you in snow. Also, wear gloves to keep your hands from freezing.

Step # 02: Finding a Location:

Follow the tips provided above in your mind when finding a place for your snow shelter. Don't choose a place that is going to get you killed eventually.

You are going to need a significant amount of snow to build your temporary accommodation in it. Therefore, final a location that already has a lot of snow instead of exerting yourself out in gathering it.

Step # 03: Selecting the Type of Shelter for You:

Selecting, which type of shelter to build, depends on the location, the amount of snow, and your physiological conditions. You can build a quinzee shelter. It takes four to five hours to make as it is a hallowed out mount. It will be warm inside.

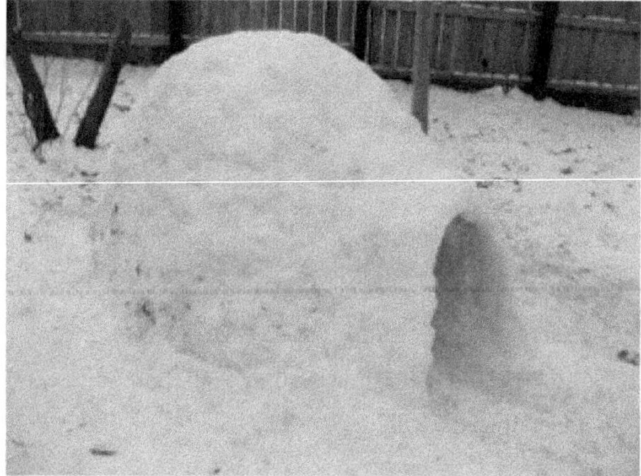

You can also dig a trench in the snow. It must be big enough to accommodate your body altogether. You can cover this trench with pine boughs, jacket, rainfly, trap, or similar. This type of shelter is just protection from the direct wind and snow. It won't be warm inside.

Step # 04: Piling Snow:

It is important when you are building a snow shelter above the ground. Gather a pile of snow of at least five to six feet height and seven to eight wide. After mounting it at a safe location, walk on it with your shoes. The snow will compress. Give it ninety minutes to two hours to settle down. It will strengthen the structure.

Step # 05: Hollowing it out:

Gather some sticks from your surroundings. They must be of eighteen inches to two feet length. Start poking these sticks in the packed snow in the form of a circle. Leave an entrance. It is ideal to keep the opening away from the wind. It will keep the insides warm.

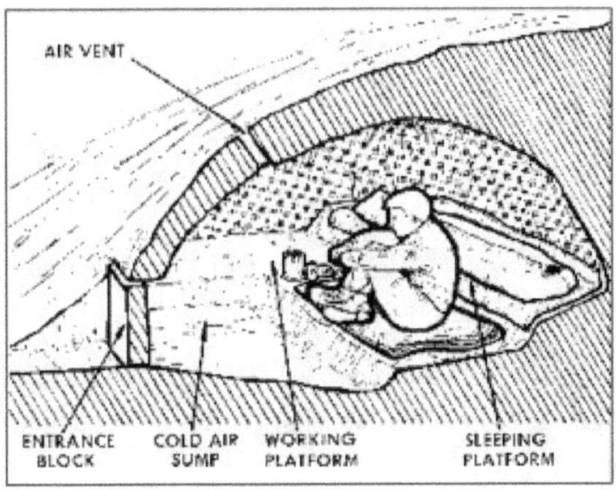

Now start digging in the snow from the center of the framework. Stop when you hit the measuring sticks forming the circle.

Step # 06: Building a Sleeping Platform:

There are two ways to create a sleeping platform within a snow shelter. The first one is to leave the sleeping area one inch higher than the ground of the shelter. Dig a trench to the entrance from under the sleeping platform. It will allow the cold air to leave the compartment as you warm it up with your body heat.

The second option is to keep the ground of the snow shelter leveled. And then build up a raised sleeping platform over it. Keep it at least one foot higher than the ground. It will help you to get the same effect on the cold air.

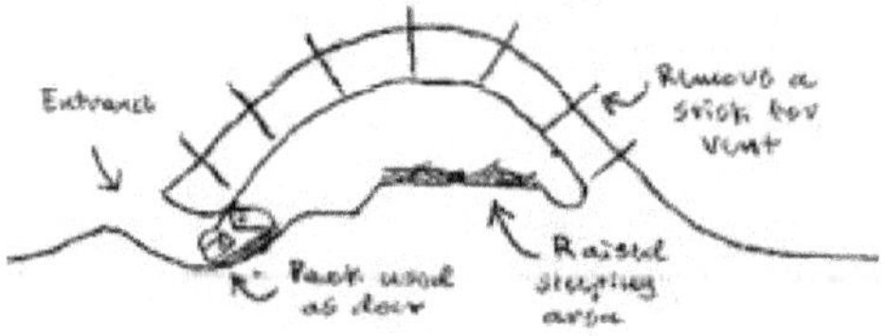

You also need to put some insulation between your body and the snow when you sleep. You can put gathered branches on your sleeping platform. You can also lay down your parachute bag and extra clothing.

Don't forget to check the breathing hole before falling asleep. Take a small branch and poke in it if it has closed by the dripping snow.

A Few Tips:

Snow naturally allows a little light to pass through it. But for lightening up the inside real bright, you need to go a few miles further. You can easily find icicles in the snowing surroundings. Gather some of them. Poke them through the roof of your temporary arrangement and they will reflect the light.

Another option is to light your candle inside a lantern or a glass jar. Then make a shelf of snow in one wall of your temporary accommodation and place it on the shelf.

It is a hustle to leave your snow shelter at night or during a snowstorm to go outside and pee. You can instead use an empty water bottle for this purpose.

If you are planning to live in the temporary accommodation for an extended period, then it is ideal to build an outdoor living area in it. It will block the cold air from entering into your sleeping compartment.

If you are lighting a candle inside, then place it on a raised platform or directly on the ground. It will keep the fire away from the melting snow.

If you want to melt the snow to convert it into drinking water, then put it in the pot with a little warm water already in it. Then heat it up on the fire.

Conclusion

Shelters are necessary to protect us from sun, rain, snow, and wind. Therefore, you only need them when the weather starts playing tricks with you. You can choose many sites to build your temporary accommodation. However, you must keep the risk factors and self-reliance opportunities of the location before finalizing one.

There are many methods and techniques through which you can build shelters robust enough to stand a storm. You can also build shelters in the wild as well as in the snow. Remember that no housing made out there in the open is safe. You can make it strong enough to stand the storms but hiding it will provide you protection and safety from both the wild animals and unfriendly passer-bys.

Survival Medicine

Introduction

If you step outside and open your eyes you will almost certainly see flowers and plants in abundance. Even if you live in the city you are likely to see window boxes and even a park or two on the way to and from work. All the plant life you seem is often taken for granted; many of us appreciate the beauty of it and may even marvel at how it reappears every year. However, what you may not appreciate is that some of these plants have the ability to literally save your life. This can be especially relevant if you are not near or cannot get to conventional medicine.

You may wonder, in the modern world, how it is possible for anyone to become isolated or cut off from conventional medicine. However, it is much easier than you think! Explorers and adventurers regularly go off the beaten tracks and search in places where very few people have been, but you would expect them to understand the risks of not being close to food supplied and medicine. However, anyone can find themselves stranded after a plane crash, shipwreck or even a long drive across the country. What begins as a small problem can quickly become a desperate survival issue. For instance, you are driving across a remote area of woodland, between two towns, unfortunately you car breaks down, as you wait safely beside the road for assistance you feel an urgent need to urinate so move deeper into the trees. A fog quickly comes down and you become disorientated. You start walking and when the fog clears you realize that you are completely lost. There is a good chance that a search party will be sent looking for you, but they may take several days to find you depending on where you have walked towards. Whilst you wait to be rescued you will need to survive.

One way in which you can increase your chances of survival is to know which herbs and plants can be eaten, which can be used as medicine and which should be avoided at all costs.   Knowing which herbs and plants can assist you will give you an edge when it comes to surviving, whether stuck in the wilderness or after the collapse of humanity! In fact, some of the herbs listed in this book can actually be taken on a regular basis to help reduce the risk of a variety of diseases. You do not need to wait until you are stranded to start taking these. The need to survive can be applied to your everyday life as herbs which can prevent you from contracting life threatening diseases are, effectively, helping you to survive!

The most important fact to take away from this book is that now is the time to learn about which herbs are good for you and can help you survive. It is no use finding yourself in that situation and wishing you had educated yourself regarding the potential of the herbs and plants around you.

Chapter 1 – Edible Plants

The list of edible plants is huge, after all the fruit and vegetables you see in your local supermarket are all grown and can be found in the wild. The majority of these products should be familiar to you already and, if you find yourself in a survival situation, you will be happy to eat these plants which you are already familiar with. If you do need to eat plants in the wild, it is important to wash them if at all possible. This will help to remove small bacteria and any small insects which could make you ill. If you are unable to find any water then you may be able to improvise, or, you may be hungry enough that the risk is worth taking.

It is important to note that this book will provide you with fifteen herbs and plants which can help save your life. There are many more which can be used to help you; your choice in the wild will be limited by the types of plant which grows in the area you are stranded in. The better your knowledge of plant life the more likely it is that you will be able to source some food to live on.

Acorns

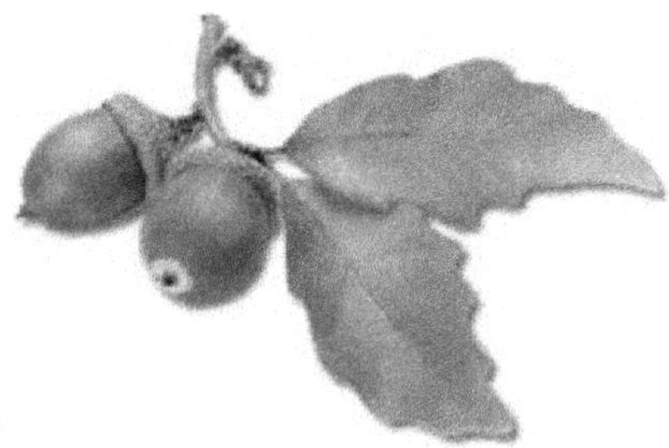

This is not something that you might usually consider eating, but they are an excellent source of protein and fat; both of which are essential to your survival. If there are oak trees in the vicinity you may find that you have a plentiful supply of acorns and this can make a huge difference to your ability to survive. Even when you are not starving it is important to eat what you can. If you do not your body will start to weaken and you will be less able to deal with simple survival tasks.

The nuts have a bitter taste and it is advisable not to consume too many of them at one time. It is also best to boil them as this will improve their flavor and make them easier to digest. The reason they taste so bitter is that they are full of tannic acid. This is not harmful but is bitter and in large quantities can give you an uncomfortable stomach.

The best method of eating acorns in the wild is to place as many as possible on a flat service as smash them with a rock. This will break their shells and you can get to the insides of them. This is the part you want to eat. You have the time it is best to soak them in warm water for a couple of hours. They are then edible; if you find they are still to bitter simply soak them for a little longer.

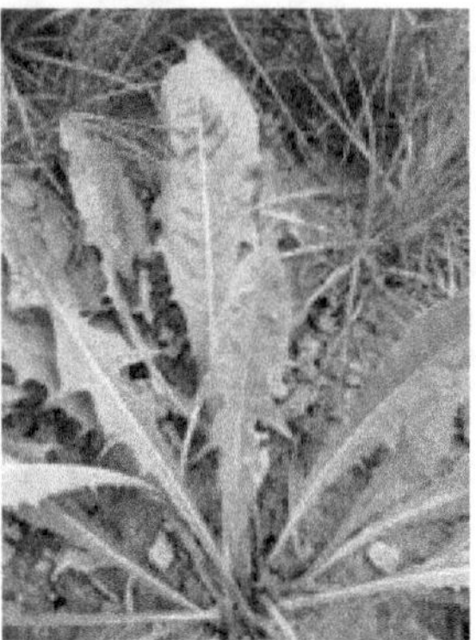

This grows almost everywhere on the planet; it is incredibly easy to recognize and surprisingly good for you. In fact, a dandelion leaf is much better for you than a standard lettuce leaf! It is known to be a plentiful supply of vitamin C, protein, fat, calcium, vitamin B, iron and even phosphorous. In fact, the humble dandelion has twelve times the amount of vitamin A that you will find in a regular lettuce leaf!

The best leaves are those which are young; although these are the smaller leaves. It is possible to eat this plant at any time of the year, although it is at its very best in the spring. It is possible to eat the leaves and even the roots if you are in a survival situation. If you are growing them at home in an attempt to add them to your diet you may wish to cut the flower heads off as early as possible; this will help the nutrition to go to the leaves and they will grow bigger. You should also protect them from the frost!

However, in the wild you can simply pull the leaves and root out of the ground and eat. It is best to wash them first; before you start looking for food you should have already found water as your body will struggle to survive for longer than a few days without water.

You can practice eating dandelion leaves at home, simply add them to a salad with your usual mixture and enjoy! It may seem like you are eating grass but this plant has a good range of nutrition which can help you stay alive.

Elderberries

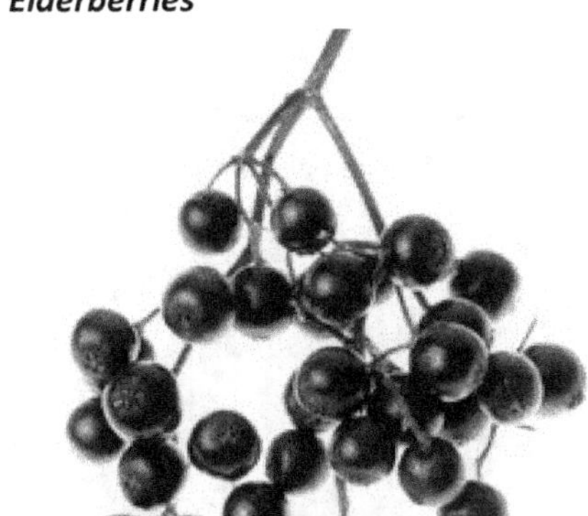

The elderberry is often overlooked when considering the variety of berries available. Traditional and better known berries, such as the blackberry or raspberry are instantly recognizable and look and taste good. In contrast the elderberry is small, very dark in color and has the potential to kill you if you do not prepare them properly!

A single shrub in the wild can easily reach ten feet and will have hundreds of berries on. It should be recognizable by its long stems with seven leaves at the end of each one. Each leaf is long and round with serrated edges. The berries are ready to be consumed in September time, obviously meaning that this survival food is seasonal. The berries are produced from the clusters of flowers which are shaped like small umbrellas. The flowers should be present in the spring and this is the best time for you to identify the plant. You will then know what you are looking for, if it becomes a necessity to eat the berries.

The berry is actually sweet and enjoyable, you can simply pick them and eat them, although be sure to check for bugs. Ideally wash them before you eat them. You should also be aware that they will turn your skin pink; although this is not a major concern when trying to survive.

Burdock

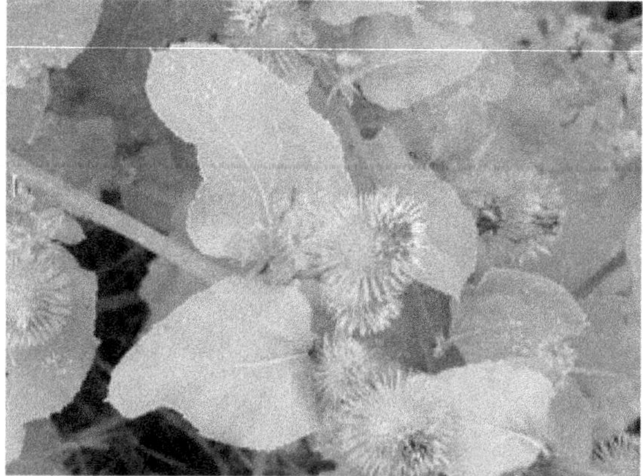

You have probably heard the words dandelion and burdock mentioned together and they are certainly both edible. The Burdock plant is medium size, towering over many weeds and comparable in size to the thistle. It also has a purple flower which bears some similarities to the standard, well known and recognized thistle. However, it does not have the large prickles of a thistle plant although the stem itself can feel prickly.

The leaves of the plant tend to be large with dips along each edge; creating an almost wrinkled effect. Originally the plant was only found in the Eastern hemisphere but it is now a common sight in many parts of the western parts of the world. It is possible to eat the leaves and the stalks, although it is necessary to peel the stalk first. You can safely eat the plant raw, however, it will taste better if it is boiled twice; this will remove the bitter taste of the leaves. It is also possible to eat the root; again you should peel it and then boil it.

Boiling may destroy some of the nutrients in any plant or herb, but, it will also help to ensure any bugs and bacteria are destroyed before you consume it. This is important as eating these plants is supposed to help you survive, not make you ill!

Cattail

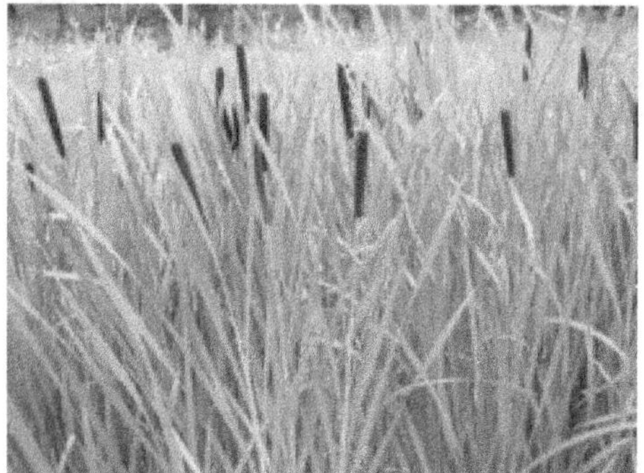

The Latin name of this plant is Typha, although it is also known as bulrush, reedmace and even punks; but you may simply refer to it as grass. It is a common sight in America, England and many other western countries. In general you will find it along the edge of the marshland; but only freshwater wetlands! This means you will need to take additional care if you are harvesting it to eat. It is possible the ground could sink under your feet, trapping you. Depending upon your location it is also possible there will be other predators in the fresh water.

If you remove the entire plant you will be able to wash the roots and eat this; it is important to wash it as you can eat this part raw. If you break the plant near the top of the root you will find that this part is the tastiest. It should appear almost completely white.

It is also possible to boil the stem and the leaves; they can then be consumed and are actually surprisingly tasty! If you are lucky enough to come across the plant in the beginning of the summer you will find that many of them have a flower which looks a little like a small corn dog. This part is also edible and can be eaten raw.

Eat it in the same way as you would a corn on the cob; in fact, it even tastes a little
like corn on the cob!

Chapter 2 – 5 Herbs Which Can Help You Stay Alive

The first chapter has dealt with plants that you can find in the wild; these are a natural food source and a valuable means of surviving whilst waiting for rescue or making your own way to civilization. However, plants are only one option; the following herbs can also help you to survive. Some of these may also help your food to be more palatable, but they will all help you to survive.

Plantain

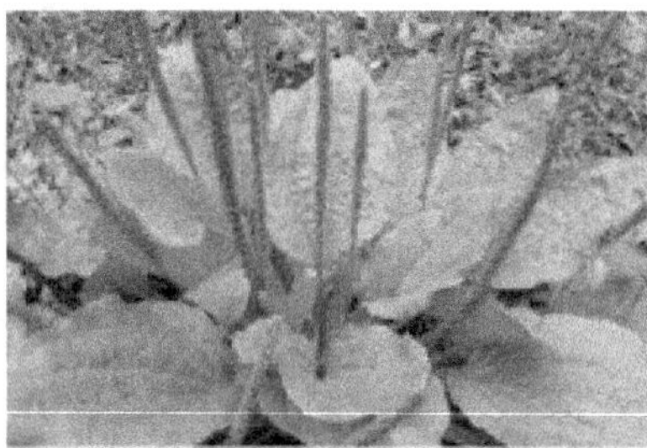

This picture shows the broad leaf variety of plantain; it is something that you are likely to have seen before as it grows almost anywhere. There is a narrow leaf version of this plant which can also be used as is just as easy to find.

The leaves can be simply picked, washed and eaten; if you combine with the nuts and berries you have already selected you will have a healthy salad which is full of valuable nutrients. Alternatively you can soak the leaf in hot water to create a tasty tea; or even use the tea to wash your skin; it is a very effective body scrub!

The herb is also known to assist with treating flu or flu like symptoms, ideally soak one whole plant in a pan of boiling water for ten minutes before drinking.

Finally, plantain is also useful for treating wounds and even burns. Smash the plant into pulp and apply this to the injured area. It will be both soothing and cleaning.

Chickweed

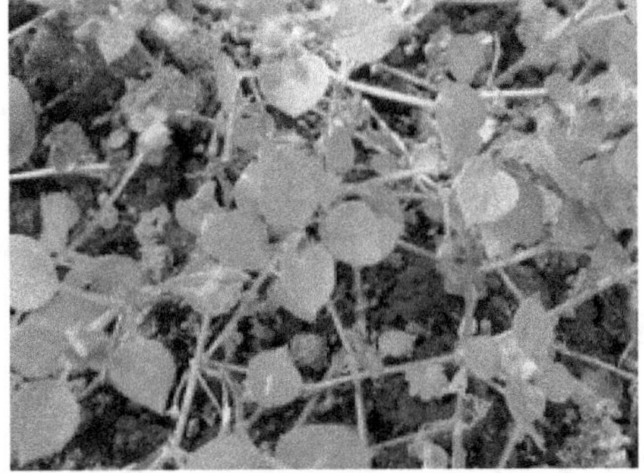

This edible plant can be called an herb or a weed. In fact it is often referred to as a weed because of the speed at which it can spread. You will probably find some of this in your garden and there will certainly be a significant quantity in the wild near you. It generally grows during the spring months although it can often be found throughout the summer months. In essence it is similar to a mild lettuce. The taste is simple, mild and yet fresh, but most importantly when surviving in the wild, it is easy to find, pick and eat. It is also full of nutrition and will help you to stay focused on the task in hand.

Again, this can be treated in much the same way as any salad leaf; you can eat it raw or mix it with any other ingredients you have to create a tasty survival dish. If you are brave enough, adding a few small grubs will really increase your protein levels and help your body to function despite the circumstances you find yourself in.

You will generally find large clumps of chickweed growing together; it will be between two inches and ten inches tall and will appear like a carpet underfoot. Chickweed is a good source of vitamin A, C and all the B's; it also provides a good mixture of metals and calcium. It has been used in the past to treat stomach upsets, circulation issues and even inflammations and blood disorders. It can also be crushed up and applied to wounds to act as an antibacterial potion.

It is worth noting that chickweed bears a startling resemblance to scarlet pimpernel. Whilst chickweed is a good source of nutrition, scarlet pimpernel is poisonous. The decisive test to confirm you have chickweed is to hold it up to the light. There will be a fine line of hairs visible on one side of the stem. It may alternate sides as it moves up or down the plant. If it does not have these hairs, do not eat it!

Wood Sorrel

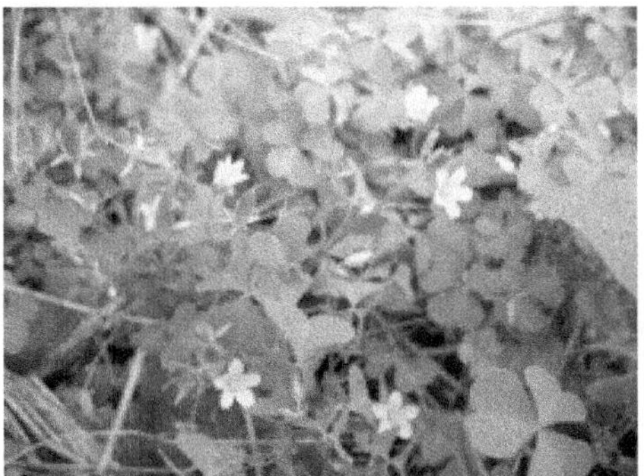

This herb is another one which is both edible and offers assistance with health issues. The plant is generally very easy to identify and, once you have sampled them the taste is not something you will forget quickly.

It looks a little like clover with the leaves appearing on opposing sides of the stem. Each set of leaves appears to be three heart shapes. Although the plant has two variants; the yellow wood sorrel and the creeping red wood sorrel, both varieties have the same yellow flowers. Each flower is like a small five pointed star, approximately half a cm wide. The stem of the plant will also be covered in microscopic hairs; you will only see these if you look exceptionally closely.

The plant can be eaten whole and raw; it tastes sour but not in an unpleasant way. In many ways you might believe you are actually eating a lemon!

It also has several medicinal qualities; it can be ground and put onto a wound to help prevent infection and to cool a burn. It can also help to regulate the kidneys and for this reason it should be avoided by anyone suffering from kidney issues. Of course, if you are trying to survive in the wild you may not be able to be too picky; in which case it should only be consumed in small amounts. It can also help to constrict your blood vessels which can be useful if you need to stop a bleed.

Another side effect of consuming too much sorrel is that it will aid the procession of food through your body and is likely to give you diarrhea; not something you want when trying to survive in the wild!

Henbit

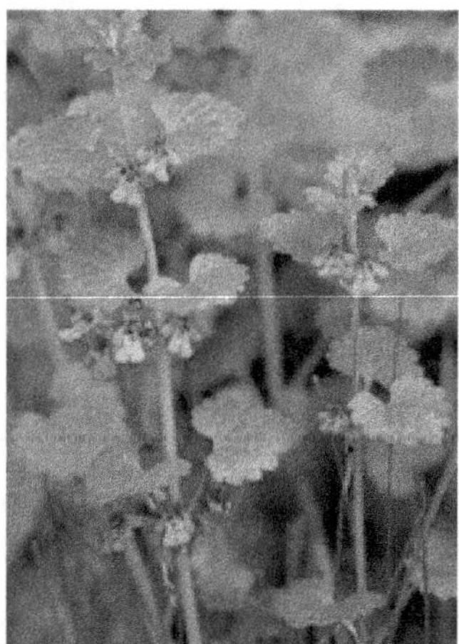

This herb is often overlooked although it can be a valuable aid when faced with a survival situation. It is very similar to purple dead nettle; however, you do not need to worry if you pick the wrong one. Dead nettle can be eaten and handled in the same as henbit, in fact, it has a similar flavor.

This herb is actually part of the mint family. It is usually recognized from the tiny flowers which are a light purple, almost pink color. The flower will appear from the middle of March until early June. The leaves are small and scallop shaped and can be eaten at any time of the year.

Despite being part of the mint family the flavor you will get from this herb is more like the taste of a lettuce leaf than mint. It is high in iron and a number of vitamins. It is also full of fiber which can help you to feel fuller for longer; something that may help you when trying to survive.

You can eat the stem and the leaves raw, or you can add them to other dishes to add a little extra flavor. It can also be soaked in hot water to make a delicious cup of tea.

Sow Thistle

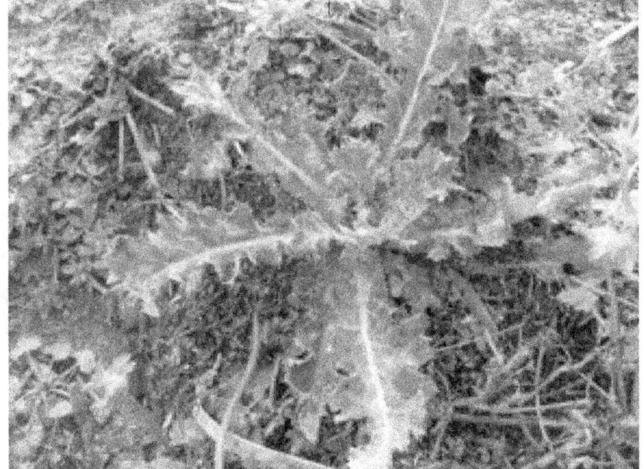

The sow thistle is usually classed as a weed, although it is, in fact, an herb. It does not look particularly appetizing as it is covered in spiny leaves. In fact, this plant has very similar properties to the dandelion, even the flower looks similar! However, you will notice the difference if you grab it quickly; the small sharp leaves will remind you of their presence.

In fact, the leaves are quite tasty. They can be eaten in the same way as a dandelion but it is essential to remove the spikes first. You can do this by pulling each one out or simply running your pocket knife around the edge of the leaf. This will cut the ends of the leaves off and leave it safe for you to eat. Even the stalks can be peeled and eaten; you will find they have a consistency similar to celery, although the taste is noticeable different.

The plant has also been acknowledged as having healing properties. It has been brewed as a tea to help remove obstructions in the urinary tract and allow comfortable urination.

As with the dandelion leaf there are a mixture of important vitamins and metals which can be obtained by eating this plant.

Chapter 3 – 5 Medicinal Herbs

Being isolated in a wilderness scenario is daunting at the best of times, but the situation can often be made much worse if you are feeling ill or have injured yourself. This can often be the case if the incident has happened suddenly and is the result of an accident. However, an injury can serious affect your ability to forage properly and may even make you a more attractive target for predators. Unfortunately once you are isolated in the wild you are much more at risk from a variety of large animals.

As well as impeding any survival attempt or your ability to travel, an injury can result in infection and consequent illness. Without antibiotics you can even find yourself succumbing to blood poisoning or other infections which are usually easily treated.

This is not a new skill; medicinal herbs have been used for generations; long before modern drugs and chemicals were created. They can be used to great effect. To ensure you are able to deal with any situation it is essential to learn which herbs can be used to treat these conditions:

Aloe Leaf

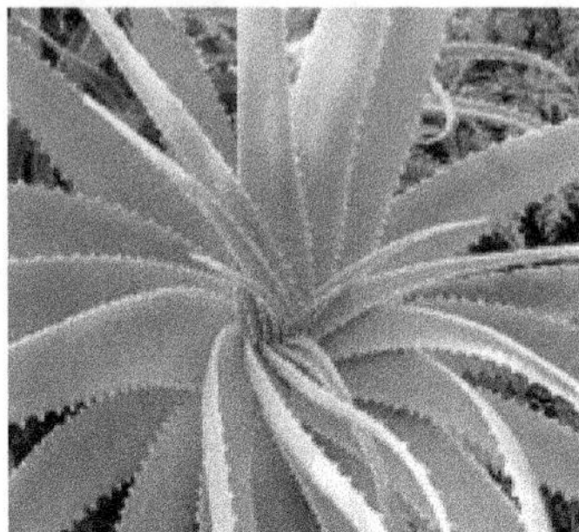

The Aloe leaf is where one of the most familiar of natural remedies comes from; aloe vera. It has been used in skin creams, sunburn lotions and even added to moisturizers and has a myriad of uses. The plant can also be found in the wild and can be a valuable benefit if you have any one of a number of injuries.

To get the valuable aloe vera lotion you will need to carefully pull a leaf of the plant and then trim all the prickles off from the leaf. You will then be able to split the leaf in half without injuring yourself further!

The exposed sap can be rubbed onto a wound, burn or even unknown skin disorders. The gel will rapidly cool and sooth the affected area allowing the body to start the healing process. It will also act as a barrier to germs and other bacteria; helping to ensure your cut does not result in an infection. It has been proven to speed up the healing process and may make the difference between you being able to forage for food or not.

Comfrey Leaf

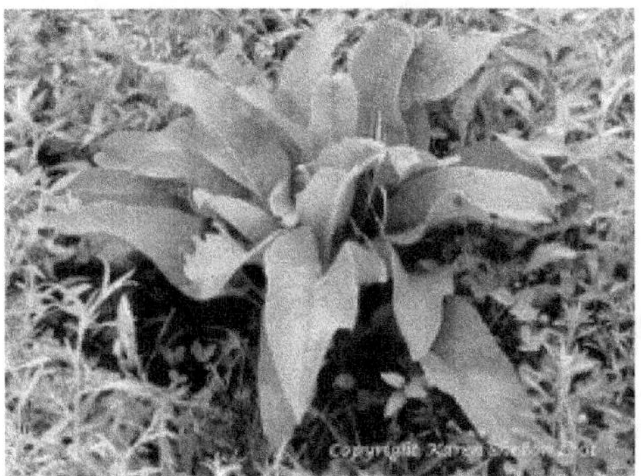

The comfrey leaf has been used in Chinese medicine for thousands of years. However, more recent research suggests that continued use of this herb internally may be toxic as it can cause damage to your liver. As you will be using this in a survival situation this is not generally an issue. It is also possible to simply use it to help with healing externally.

The leaf has been shown to help stop bleeding and can even encourage your tissues to regenerate; speeding the time it takes for your body to repair itself. The leaves can be ground into a paste and then applied to the skin, either directly to a cut or over the site of a fractured bone. It will soak into the body and help your injured bone heal. It is even effective if you apply it to muscles and tendons which you have pulled or strained.

It is important to note that the comfrey leaf is incredibly fast acting. Any cut will be sealed in moments; effectively trapping any dirt or bacteria in the wound. You must be certain the wound is clean before you seal it with this herb. If it is still bleeding then this is a good sign that the wound is clean as any debris or bacteria are likely to be carried out with the blood.

St. John's Wort

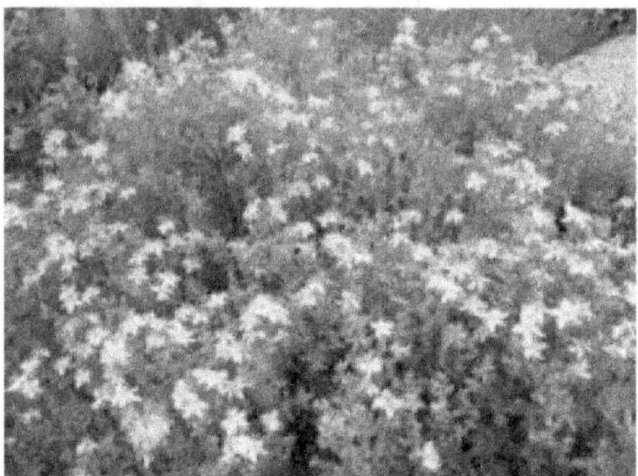

This is another natural herb which is present in a wide variety of over the counter products. It can even be bought in liquid form. The plant grows almost anywhere, it will quickly spread and cover any spare land with its green stems and bright yellow flowers. If left, they will grow to waist height relatively quickly.

The best part to use when in the wild is the flower bud, not the flower itself. This can be crushed and it will produce a liquid which is red, bordering on purple. This liquid can then be applied directly to an injured area to provide plain relief. In fact St. John's Wort is a very effective pain reliever as it targets the nerves directly. It will actively encourage your nerves to start healing and reduce the pain in the process.

It is possible to harvest the buds in the summer and mix them with olive oil which can then be drunk to assist with pain killing. However, this is unlikely to be an option in the wild.

An additional benefit of St. John's Wort is that it is naturally an anti-depressant. This may seem trivial but anything which can help; to keep your spirits up in a survival situation will be of benefit!

Yarrow

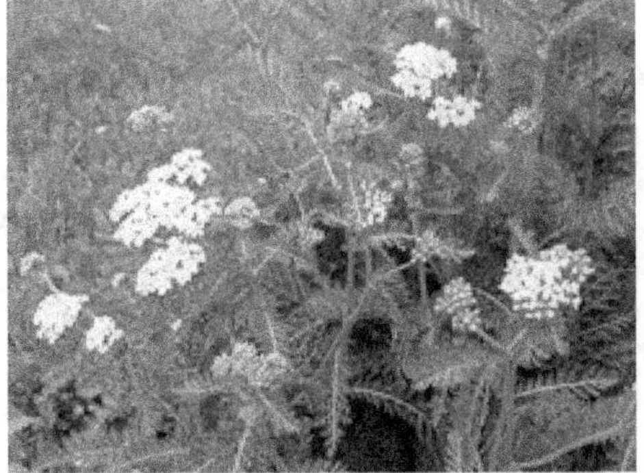

This plant can be found in many parts of the world and is easy to distinguish thanks to its fern like leaves and clusters of white flowers. It is an exceptionally good way of stopping bleeding; this will allow you to treat your wound and start recovering. Blood will also attract predators so it is advisable to move on as soon as you have stopped the bleeding.

You can make a paste from the flowers by crushing them; between two rocks or even between your fingers. The paste can be applied directly to a wound to stop the bleeding.

It has also been used to make tea by brewing in hot water for a minimum of five minutes. The tea is effective at treating colds, fevers and a range of digestive problems. It should not be taken over an extended period of time as it can be toxic.

Jewelweed

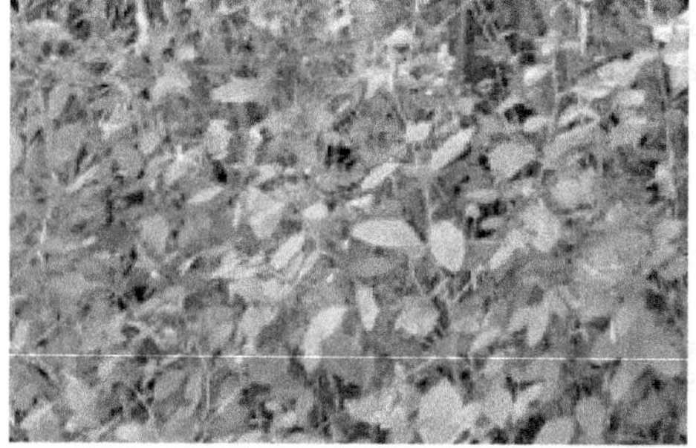

This plant has tall slim stems with a flower hanging off the top; in many ways it has the appearance of a jewel hanging on a necklace; in fact, this I how the plant got its name. It has been used for many years to treat outbreaks of poison ivy, although it is effective against almost any kind of plant based rash. To use this in the wild you will need to squeeze or crush the stem and even the leaves; this will produce a clear liquid which can be used to gently rub on the affected area. The soothing effects of this plant will be felt almost immediately; allowing you to focus on more important survival tasks.

The extract from this plant is also effective when used to treat bruises, burns and even cuts. It has even been effective at taking away the soreness of an insect bite; something which could prove very valuable when in the wilderness.

It is also interesting to note that the jewelweed is often found growing near poison ivy; as though nature has provided the cure ready for you!

Conclusion

This book has merely touched on the number of herbs and plants which are available in the wild and can be used to aid survival. There are many more. However, it is important to study these plants now and be certain you know what you are looking at. There are many plants which can benefit your health but which look very similar to ones which will make you ill, or even kill you. By studying these plants now you will have no issue when needing them to survive.

It is quite possible that you will have heard it said that humans can go for weeks and sometimes even months without food, providing they have water. If you have no water you will be unlikely to survive longer than three or five days. This means that if you are in a survival situation water and shelter are the most important things.

But, once you have found these, it remains an important goal to source food. If you do not your body will go into fasting mode, you will immediately notice the affect of this and will have less energy and less motivation. Eating even small amounts of food per day will keep your body from moving into this mode and provide important nutritional benefit. Perhaps even more importantly will be the psychological and emotional effect. Being able to source food and locate plants to help treat any injuries will provide you with a mental lift. You will know it is possible to survive in the wilderness; instead of wondering if you will ever be rescued or if you will die alone in the wilderness, you will be considering the best plan to take you back to civilization. Water and shelter are essential physical needs; food is the essential emotional lift which will get you home.

Of course, there are plenty of plants which will harm you and the golden rule is if you are not sure to leave them alone. However, if your hunger increases and you have not had any success finding the plants and herbs you do know about then it is important to avoid any plant which displays the following symptoms:

- Colored sap; in general a plant with clear sap will be safe to eat; although wherever possible you should wash or boil it first.

- Thorny or spiky plants are usually dangerous; this is nature's way of warning people and animals to stay away from them. This is not always true but if you are unfamiliar with a specific plant it is best to err on the side of caution.

- Taste; ideally you should try as many of the plants you are likely to encounter and may need to rely on before you go on a trip. If you are sampling plants it is best to ensure your palate is clear first. This will ensure you obtain the full flavor. The benefit of doing this now is that if you are stuck in the wild you will be able to taste a very small part of a plant and know whether it tastes like it should. If it does not then you should not eat it.

- Mushrooms are exceptionally hard to calculate whether they are okay to eat or not. There are many different species and some of the nicest ones look very similar to some of the deadliest ones! If you do find mushrooms and you believe they are edible it is best to try a small piece and then wait, ideally for twenty four hours, before you have any more.

Knowing which plants and herbs have medicinal properties can be as important as food, any injury you receive in the wild will be far worse than one in a civilized area simply because you will not have access to medical care. There are plants which can stop the bleeding, provide pain relief and even act as an antiseptic; providing you know what you are looking for.

There is a marked increase in the ability to live off the land and an abundance of information. Once you have mastered the basics illustrated in this book you will be able to advance your learning; it is a fascinating subject!

Emergency Drinking Water Storage

Introduction: Are We Running out of Water?

I remember doomsayers warning us years ago that water would one day run out and most of us would just be out of luck left to bake in the sun. These were the same folks that routinely told us that the hole in the ozone layer (Apparently caused by hairspray bottles; thanks a lot 80's hairstyle designs!) would grow so large that it would envelope the entire planet by 2005.

Well newsflash folks! It's now 2016 and nobody even mentions the ozone layer anymore. And for much the same reason, no one tries to scare us over the possibility of "wars over water" either. Because the truth is, the Earth's supply of water is so abundant—71% of the Earth is covered in it—we haven't even tapped into half of it yet! This then brings us to what is really at stake in our quest for H_2O, because it is not a matter of water supply that is the problem, it is a matter of access.

Even in those remote parts of the world where you hear of people struggling to drink from dwindling dirty water supplies, the reason for their struggle is because they just haven't found the reserves of water that still remain locked under their feet. And the statistics are staggering about 1 billion people in the world at any given time do not have any means of storing safe drinking water.

But in many of these same regions, after a proper survey of the land, it just takes digging a few feet into the ground to produce a well that will supply water almost indefinitely for years to come. That can be stored away for the use of future generations of people. So yes, once again, the water is there, we just have to find it, and after we find it we have to know how to store it. This book strives to show you just how you can not only find water, but store it and keep it always at the ready just in case the spit hits the fan!

Chapter 1: How to Prep Your Water

Before we even get into different modes and methods of storing water we need to take the time to discuss how we can make sure that the water we store is safe for us to drink. And while most tap water and bottled water purchased from your grocery store shouldn't cause you a problem, just in case you are using water from other less secure sources—as we will highlight later in this book—let's delve into just how you can filter and purify water regardless of where you might get it.

The oldest method of purifying water is to simply boil it. Boiling water should get rid of most contaminants, set the water to a full boil for about 1 minute and most harmful organisms will die. Next to boiling water, filters are a great tool to use as well. The best store bought filters have the title of "purification grade" and they will also most likely have what is known as "iodine impregnated" resin beads that release a cleansing iodine formula into the water as it is simultaneously filtered by the apparatus.

And for all you DIY enthusiasts out there, if you don't have a store bought filter, you can always make one of your own from scratch. All you really need to make a good filtering mechanism is a 2 liter plastic soda bottle and a coffee filter. Just cut open the bottom of the plastic bottle and then place the coffee filter over the opening. Now secure the filter to the bottom of the 2 liter with a rubber band or a piece of tight rope or twine.

This is your basic filtering apparatus, as you have probably guessed, to use the device you will simply pour the water you wish to filter through the top opening of the 2 liter and then let it sift through the coffee filter tied to the bottom of the bottle, leaving the unsafe sediment and other elements safely in the plastic bottle. You can filter your water like this over a large bowl or other wide mouthed container and then seal the filtered water up after you are done.

Another option for you to make your water drinkable is to drop in a couple of chlorine tablets. Working on the same premise as the chlorinated water of a swimming pool, these powerful agents will quickly clean out your water, the only trouble is, if you remember what it was like when you accidentally swallowed a mouthful of swimming pool water, it isn't always that pleasant. But regardless, these methods of prepping your water just might save your life.

Chapter 2: Using Your Home's Ready Made Containers

Some of the best places to store our water may be right in the structure of our very home. Modern architecture is replete with water based systems all throughout the frame of the house. These places are natural repositories for the water that you receive on a daily basis from the worn out, old infrastructure, known as a grid.

This water is pumped in to us every single day, filling up these ready made containers ensconced within the walls, floorboards, plumbing and heating systems in our homes. It's already there, so we might as well attempt to make use of them. So if all of the civil infrastructures start falling apart all around you, start looking toward these artificial reservoirs conveniently built right into your home and start tapping into these naturally occurring containers lodged deep within your house.

The Water Heater

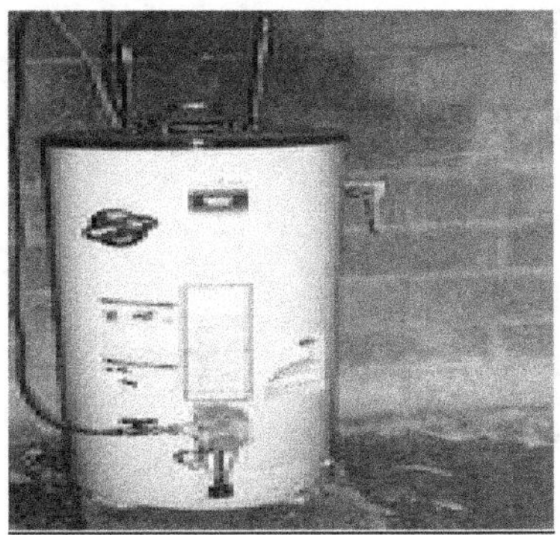

The first naturally occurring, built-in water container for your home that we should consider is that of the water heater. Just consider the possibilities, you have a large upright cylinder, a water tank, strategically placed right in the middle of your house, specifically designed to hold heated water; it certainly sounds like a water container to me. In order to safely access this water all you have to do is go to your circuit breaker and switch the power off, and then open the vent on your heater and then pull on the lever that releases the spigot and let your water come pouring out.

You can then fill up as many additional jugs up with this precious water resource as much as you want. You should be able to produce several gallons from most standard water heaters. Just one word of caution; be sure to filter the water before you start drinking it, since water heaters tend to have sediment and other debris stored in them. Most of this material is easy to see though, and will quickly float to the top, making it a fairly easy task to filter them out from the rest the water.

Household Pipes

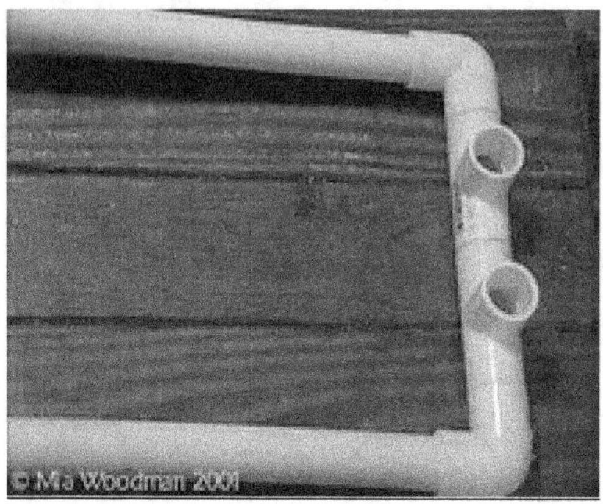

Yes the very pipes in your home carry an abundance of water and if you could only learn to slow their flow you will be able to store plenty of it within those valves. To seal the water within your pipes simply turn off your main water line. To some that might seem counterproductive since the whole purpose of the exercise is to be able to store water. But this is not the case, in a true emergency such as a flood or hurricane tap water stations can become quickly compromised, if you have adequate time however, and you shut off your water line ahead of the disaster you should be able to prevent contamination.

With most pipes having a capacity that reaches into the gallons, you should be able to save a lot of unaffected water in your pipes and store it up for later use. Once the water is trapped in your pipes you can store it there almost indefinitely. When you would like to use the water simply turn on your faucet like you normally would and after a little bit of air releases, your stored water should come pouring out of the faucet. After you get the water flowing, make sure that you collect as much of this stored H2O as you can, because by all accounts the typical household should have many gallons of water stored right in their pipes.

The Bathroom Toilet

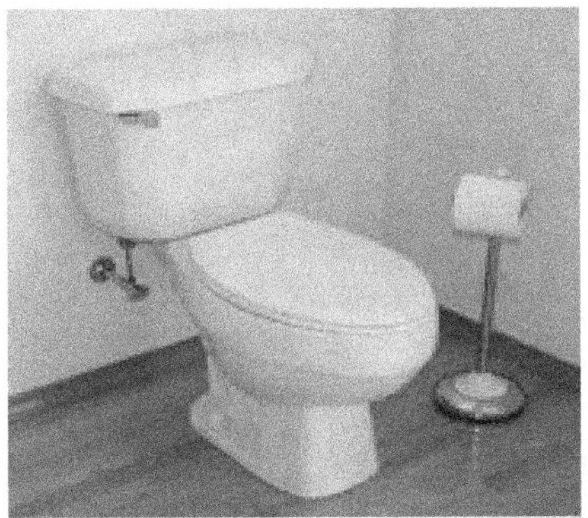

Yes, I fully realize that this is probably one of the going to be one of the grossest things that you ever heard of. But if it makes you feel any better I am not talking about storing water in your toilet bowl. When I talk about storing drinking water in your toilet I am referring to the tank of your toilet. Because while the water in your toilet bowl is no doubt filled with all kinds of nasty critters, by all accounts, the water in the tank of your toilet should be fairly safe for consumption.

In order to trap this water, just like you did for your pipes, shut off your water line, now just keep people from flushing the toilet and you will have drinkable water stored right in the tank of your toilet ready for you to transfer it to other more reliable household containers. Yes, even though it doesn't sound very appetizing to store your drinking water in the back of your toilet tank, in the end if it can help save lives during an emergency, it will be worth it.

The Bathtub

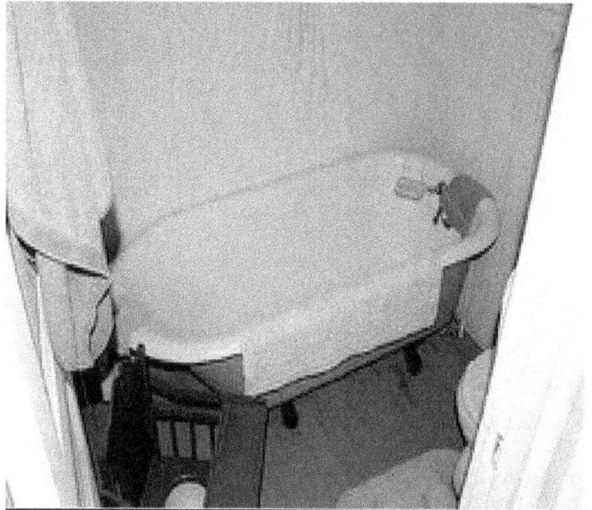

A little better than the toilet, but it still may be a little bit hard to get used to the idea of storing drinking water in the place where you normally bathe. And you have valid reason to be a bit concerned because any water stored in a bathtub will no doubt be susceptible to the months of caked on bacteria from peoples feet (and other body parts that will remain unmentionable) as they get in and out of the tub.

Not only that, an even worse threat that a bathtub may pose to water are the chemicals that you used the last time that you tried to clean out your bathtub. These chemical agents can remain on the surface of a tub for months at a time. But don't worry because this dilemma can easily be solved by using a homemade filter, boiling the water, or using chlorine tablets as discussed in the previous chapter. These precautionary measures are required for this DIY storage unit, and if done properly it should do the trick in sterilizing this water for further use.

So having that said, if you have enough notice, before the storm (or whatever the crisis may be) comes along, just fill up your bathtub like you normally would with the drain stopper in place to secure the water. The best thing about this bathtub water is its sheer storage capacity because the average bathtub can store up to 100 gallons of water. In a true crisis situation, that massive surplus of H2O could wind up saving your life.

Household Sinks

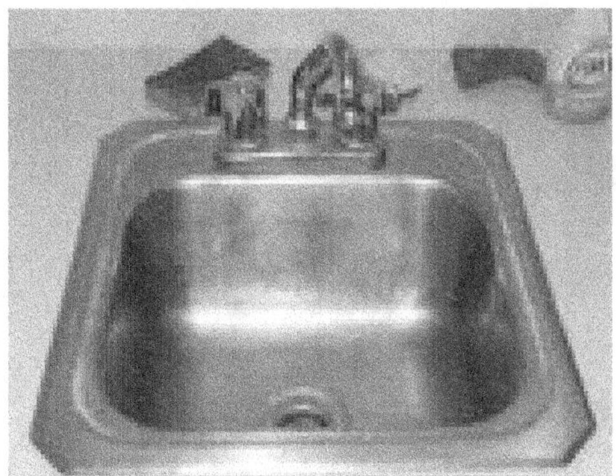

Just like the bathtub option mentioned above, before an emergency situation erupts, fill up your sinks with as much water as you can and them stop up by covering the drain. This water should actually be in fairly good shape, but you should still boil it or otherwise sterilize it before drinking it nonetheless.

To transfer this water just use a small to medium sized water bottle and put it down to the bottom of the sink letting it slowly fill with water. Empty store bought bottled water containers work just fine for this, just place them down to the bottom and you will see and hear the water bubbling as the bottle collects this liquid resource.

Rain Barrel

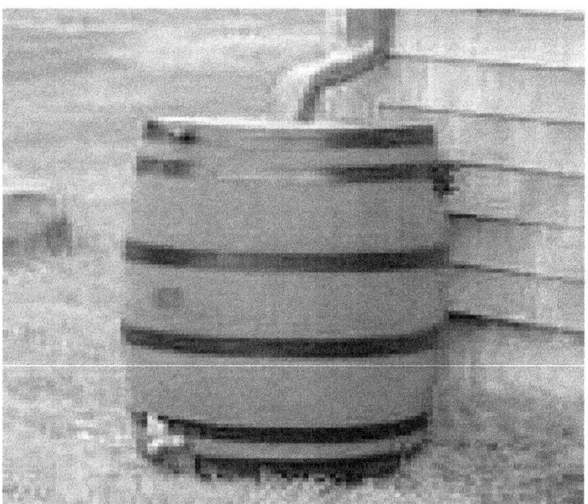

Now for our last entry into the world of naturally occurring household storage units you may find your self scratching your head with this one. Because yes, while I admit that a rain barrel is not an immediately imbedded storage unit in the home, I am going to include it anyway because it can work as a necessary tool to get water from one of the ready made storage containers already attached to your house.

And in this case the ready made storage container that I am referring to is the gutters of your home. These gutters are designed to allow rain to collect inside them, usually this collected water then moves on to slide down the gutter back to the ground below. But what if we could intercept this water resource before it hits the ground?

This is where are rain barrel comes in, because just as the name implies, "Rain Barrels" are meant to collect rain, safely storing them within their structure for later use. Having that said, just take one of these bad boys and strategically place it right under the bottom of one of your home's gutter pipes and you will quickly see the barrel fill up with all of the rain's runoff as the water flows through the gutter of your home.

In that sense the Rain Barrel is more of the mode of transfer and the gutter is the actual storage unit readily built into your home. But either way you look at it, it is a great idea that will allow you to store up even more water during an emergency. After you collect your water however, just like all of the other examples, make sure you filter or otherwise sanitize your rainwater as well.

Chapter 3: Storing Water in Auxiliary Household Containers

After covering some of the built in storage units that can be found throughout the home, in this chapter we are going to focus on using additional auxiliary containers such as jugs and bottles that you can use to store surplus water in the home. We all have them lying around somewhere taking up space, so we might as well stock up on them so we can continue on our prepping journey. This chapter highlights some of the best household containers for long term water storage, and how you should use them.

2 Liter Soda Bottles

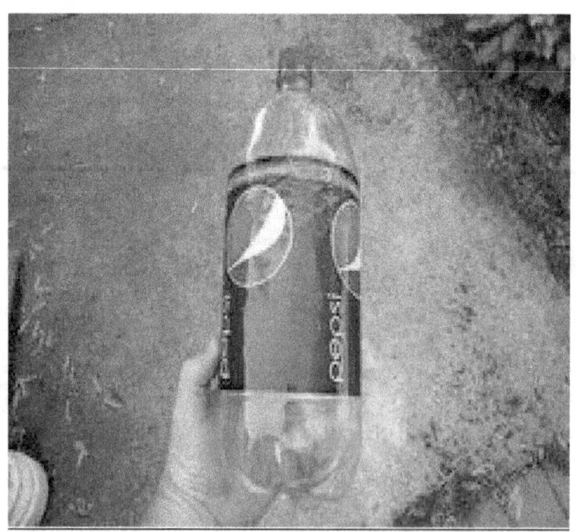

These are the kinds of containers that we can all relate to; they are ubiquitous and no doubt scattered throughout countless households all over the world. In order to store your water in these 2 liter soda bottles, first rinse and wash the containers with dish soap and water. I usually put the soap down in the bottom, fill the bottle halfway with water, then shake it as hard as I can for a few minutes and let the centrifugal forces do the rest.

Once you have washed out these containers in this manner simply put them out to dry. I find that a sunny windowsill does a great job at thoroughly drying out the bottles; I've also used hair dryers before to directly dry them out. After the bottles are dry, then just fill these guys up with clear water and save them for later when you might really need them.

Milk Jugs

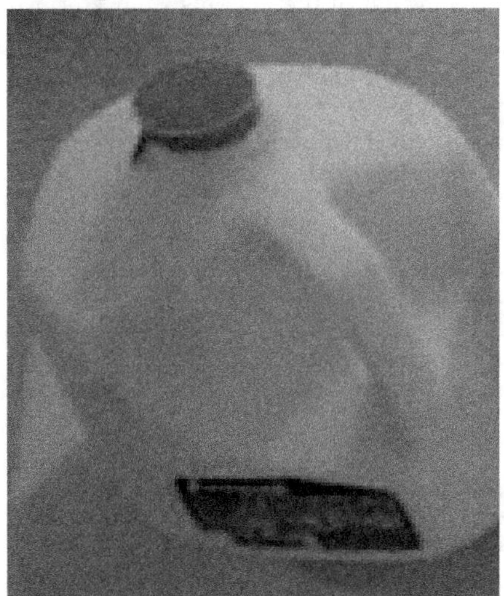

Milk Jugs can carry a full gallon of water, and since we typically gauge our daily water consumption in the gallons it makes for an ideal means of mass storage. Just make sure you clean out the container. Because the fact is, something that is used to contain milk, posing a much greater risk of contamination than a bottle that just housed a few drops of Coca-Cola.

So yes, anything that dairy products were once a part of needs to be even more thoroughly cleaned, since remnants of spoiled milk will quickly contaminate your water supply. On milk containers I usually use a few methods of cleaning them out, I typically take a high power hose to its insides to thoroughly knock out any clinging milky remnants, but if you don't have a hose you can also use the sprayer commonly attached to most kitchen sinks.

After I've thoroughly sprayed the milk jug down I then put in my cleaning solution and allow it to soak inside the plastic for a good 2-3 hours. I then pour out the cleaning solution and start spraying the insides of the milk jug again to rinse it out. The whole process is basically just a big, "Rinse, Wash, and Repeat". But either way, once you clean all of those remnants out of the container and just fill it up, seal it with a lid and put it away in storage and you have yet another gallon of water that you can depend upon in an emergency.

Glass Jars

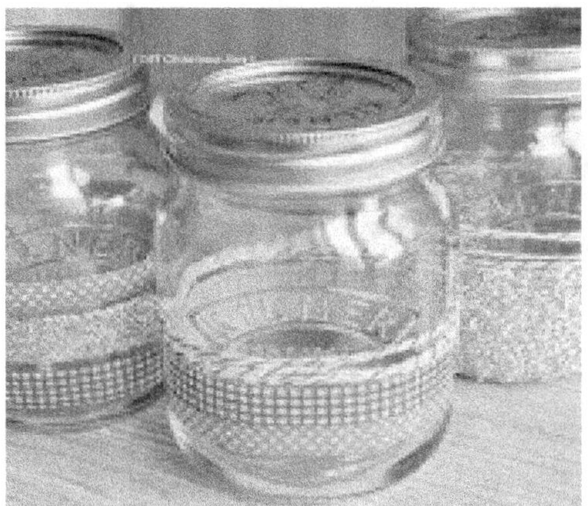

Glass jars are a durable container and can be used to store water for a practically indefinite amount of time. By using quart sized glass jars you can store plenty of water and then be able to neatly stack them up in your cupboards and cabinets. When you begin filling your jars with water just make sure that you leave about one inch of space at the top so that your water has room for expansion. Once you have done this, seal the jar shut with your lid. You can then boil the jars in a tub or use a steamer canner to seal them. Boiling time for these jars should take about 30 minutes.

Polyethylene Barrels

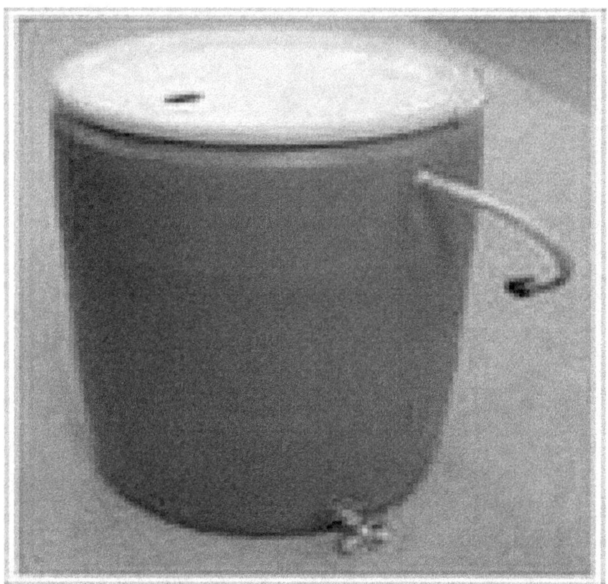

Much like the rain barrels mentioned earlier in this book, polyethylene barrels are durable and are extremely useful for storing large amounts of water. You can find these barrels at most hardware and food suppliers. One thing to keep in mind about these containers however is that since they store such a large amount of water (up to 55 gallons) you need to have a permanent place to store the barrel itself, since it will be so difficult to move later on.

And if you really do have to move a fully loaded polyethylene barrel you will undoubtedly need some mechanical assistance such as a lifting device. But once you have these containers placed in the right spot, they can work as a constant resource for you during your time of need.

Coolers

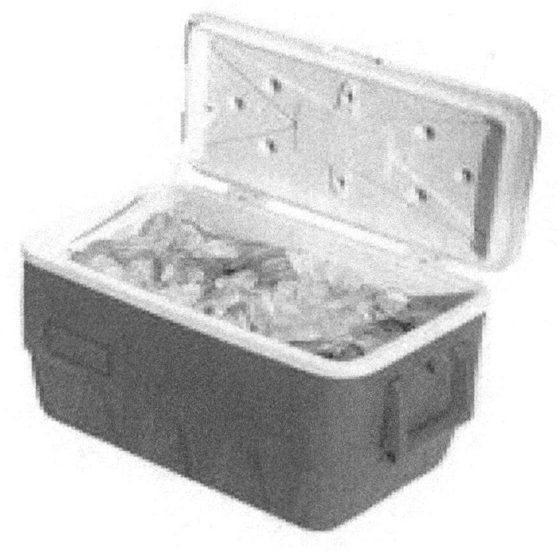

Conventional coolers (such as the picnic variety) are another great option to store potable drinking water. As with everything else, just make sure you sanitize your cooler and clean it out. Because after months of family picnics and other excursions, the good old cooler probably has gotten a bit dirty. Once this icon of family fun is clean however, just fill that buddy up with water, close the lid and you are good to go. Coolers are convenient as a water storage apparatus because they are easy to carry. Just grab the handle of this water supply and take it to the picnic!

Store Bought Bottled Water

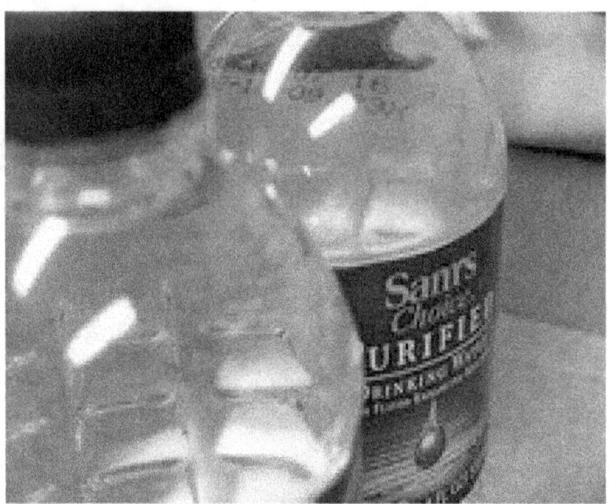

These are great bought from the store just as they are. These water bottles are conveniently designed with long term water storage in mind. You can buy several packages of 36 packs of bottled water and then stack them up and store them in right in your garage or pantry.

Buy 7 or 8 of these and it should be enough to last you through the month. And then as an added bonus save the all your containers so that once you've drank up all of the store bought water you can then refill your plastic bottles with additional water once again. In my humble opinion it would never hurt to have some store bought packs of water laying around just in case of an emergency.

I know that some preppers may turn their nose at this, and might think that using store bought water bottles is somehow some kind of a cop out when it comes to

DIY survival prep—but hey—there are no rules to survival. And whether you are drinking from pristine "Ice Mountain" store bought water bottles, or drinking out of a toilet, the fact that you are surviving and able to drink at all, is what really matters in the end!

Chapter 4: Ingenious Ways to Store Water Outside

The house is a good place to store water and the most obvious choice, but maybe you don't want to be so obvious, and for whatever reason you would rather be a little bit more discreet as to where you stockpile your supply of water. Well then, have you thought about storing your water in the great outdoors? If worse came to worse; societal shutdown, alien invasion, or zombie apocalypse.

Maybe you shouldn't keep all your water stocked up in plain sight where all those thirsty zombies and aliens might see them! (Or for that matter demanding neighbors.) And so it is with the pressures of societal meltdown during a crisis in mind, that in this chapter we are going to give you a quick rundown of some of the best places and containers in which you can store your stockpile of water safely outside of your home.

Large Trash Bags

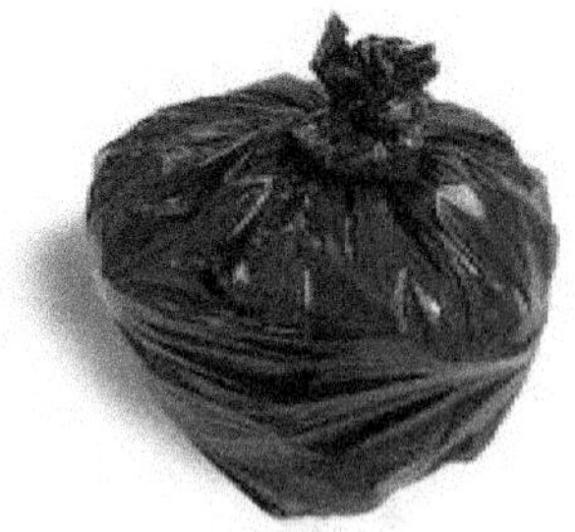

I know this one may seem a little bit odd, but if you are worried about someone else coming along and snatching up your vital supply of water, a trash bag may be one of the best ways to conceal your stash of H2O. No one would think to look in a trash bag for water right? That's the whole point. So before the spit hits the fan go ahead and grab up a large (and durable) heavy duty trash bag, make sure it is clean and there are no holes or tears in the body of the bag and then fill it up with water.

Now take a piece of rope or twine and seal that trash bag up as tight as you can. Once you have this bag sealed up you have a few options with what you could do with it, you could partially conceal it in a pile of leaves, or leave it near a trashcan, hiding it in plain sight. Or you could even bury the bag in a safe spot so you know that it will be safe and un-tampered with by the time you actually need to use it. Converting a trash bag into a water depository is a great way to conceal fresh water.

Old Washing Machine

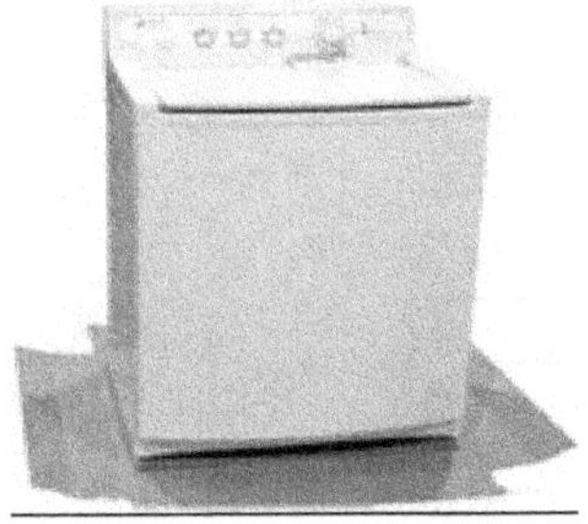

If you have a garage like mine which is a wasteland of old junk, then you could probably get away with a old piece of junk washer sitting in plain sight being used as a water tank. Naturally, as a device meant to cycle and wash load after load of clothing, washing machines have a high capacity when it comes to storing water. Several gallons can be stored up, right in the body of the machine.

Another good thing about using a washing machine as a water storage unit is the fact of how well the device can seal itself up. Once you shut the lid down it should be airtight, making sure that nothing gets in and nothing gets out. In a washing machine your water should be just as safe as it would be closed up in a water bottle. Just try your best to clean out the washer and then just fill it up and shut the lid. Utilizing a bit of up-cycling hackery you can make a great water tank out of that junky old washer.

Water Well

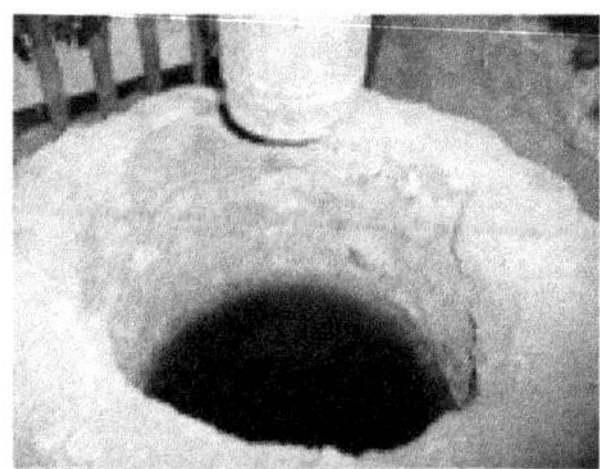

This method actually constitutes both a way to get water and a way to store it, since digging a well is tapping into the water that is already stored outside your door, deep down in the earth. In order to reach this underground water supply you will need to dig about 30 feet deep. Once you dig out a 20 foot hole you need to stabilize this entry point by lining the walls with either concrete or gravel rocks. After you have done this create a cap to cover up the hole and prevent contamination.

When you are ready to retrieve your water just take a solid wooden, metal, or even plastic bucket and tie a rope around its handle, now just hurl that thing down the well until it starts lapping up water and then like you're a fisherman reeling in the big one, just pull that bucket up, and you will have the freshest water you could ever get, stored right there in the best storage container ever conceived; the ground under your feet!

Conclusion: The Ultimate Storage Unit

As we touched upon in the introduction of this book, for many years we were fed the false claim that we would soon run out of water, this has been effectively proven false and those that perpetuate such wild claims are suffering from a gross misunderstanding of how our world and even the entire universe really works. It is true that our planet in its goldilocks zone is fairly lucky to be inundated with such large amounts of free flowing surface water; the planetary feature that has become so iconic from space photo's, giving our world a fitting new nickname as the "blue planet".

But even so, science has inherently proven that water is by no means unique to Earth. Water itself is merely a byproduct of star formation in the cosmos. Because when a star (sun) forms its formation disk sends out a large plume of gas and dust that rides the solar wind. At their heart stars are powerful nuclear furnaces, and their formation is dynamic, sending shockwaves that then heat and compress this escaping plume of gas. Well ladies and gentlemen, I hate to break it to you, but it is this cloud of interstellar gas that our water actually comes from!

Indicating that water is not unique to Earth and in no way originated from Earth; it is simply a routine byproduct that occurs after one of billions upon billions of stars are born. Water is literally, just out there, floating around in space! So as you can see, contrary to what some have claimed, water is actually a quite common element that has been scattered all throughout all of creation.

But even though water is not unique to Earth, what does make our little blue planet unique is the mean by which our world *stores water*. Because as of right now, although the element that makes up water seem quite common, no other planetary body that we know of, stores water as well as ours. At least at this moment in time, the Earth could be said to be the best known water container in the universe.

While other planets such as Venus and Mars are miserable failures at holding water (too hot or too cold to retain it) the Earth is just right. And unlike the doomsday predictors who said we may run out of water because of our wasteful habits, no matter how wasteful we may be, our resourceful planet is perfectly efficient at recycling all of its water, including the 96.5 % found in the planet's seas and oceans, the 1.7% in groundwater, the 1.7% in glaciers, the 0.0001% in the atmosphere and even the 0.003% resides within the bodies of all of Earth's biological organisms (like me and you).

All this water, as wasteful as we think we are, all of it is accounted for. None of Earth's water is just thrown away, it doesn't just get tossed off the planet into the vacuum of space, in the end none of it is going anywhere, because as soon as it rises up into the atmosphere as water vapor, it hits the cold jet stream which freezes it and causes it to fall back to the earth as rain and snow. Even the water in our own bodies ultimately doesn't disappear, it may not be pleasant to think about it, but yes, even urine is eventually recycled and used once again by the Earth's natural processes.

So in closing, I would just like for you to know that Earth has had quite a monopoly on these water based compounds within our galactic neighborhood for the past 4 billion years and counting. And despite what you may have heard and what the crazed climate change fanatics may tell you, the insignificant little rumblings of the small little band of creatures called humans (who only showed up about 500,000 years ago) are not going to change that monopoly on water storage anytime soon. Making our wonderful Earth itself, the ultimate in water storage capacity; our planet is the ultimate storage unit.

FREE Bonus Reminder

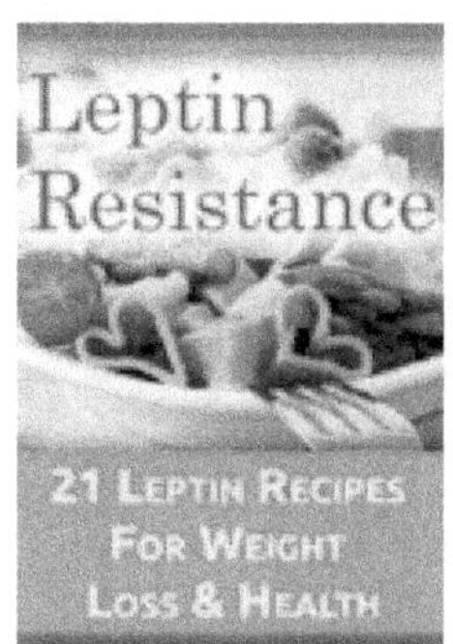

If you have not grabbed it yet, please go ahead and download your special bonus report *"Leptin Resistance. 21 Leptin Recipes For Weight Loss & Healthy Living"*.

Simply Click the Button Below

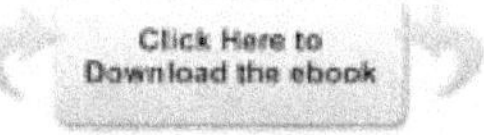

OR **Go to This Page**

http://easyweightlossway.com/free/

BONUS #2: More Free & Discounted Books

Do you want to receive more Free & Discounted Books?

We have a mailing list where we send out our new Books when they go free or with a discount on Kindle. Click on the link below to sign up for Free & Discount Book Promotions.

=> Sign Up for Free & Discount Book Promotions <=

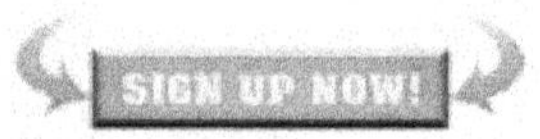

OR Go to this URL

http://zbit.ly/1WBb1Ek